# KETTLEBELL EXERCISE ENCYCLOPEDIA

Kettlebell exercises and variations in one handy book with detailed photos.

**VOLUME 4/5:** Squat, Swing, Windmill

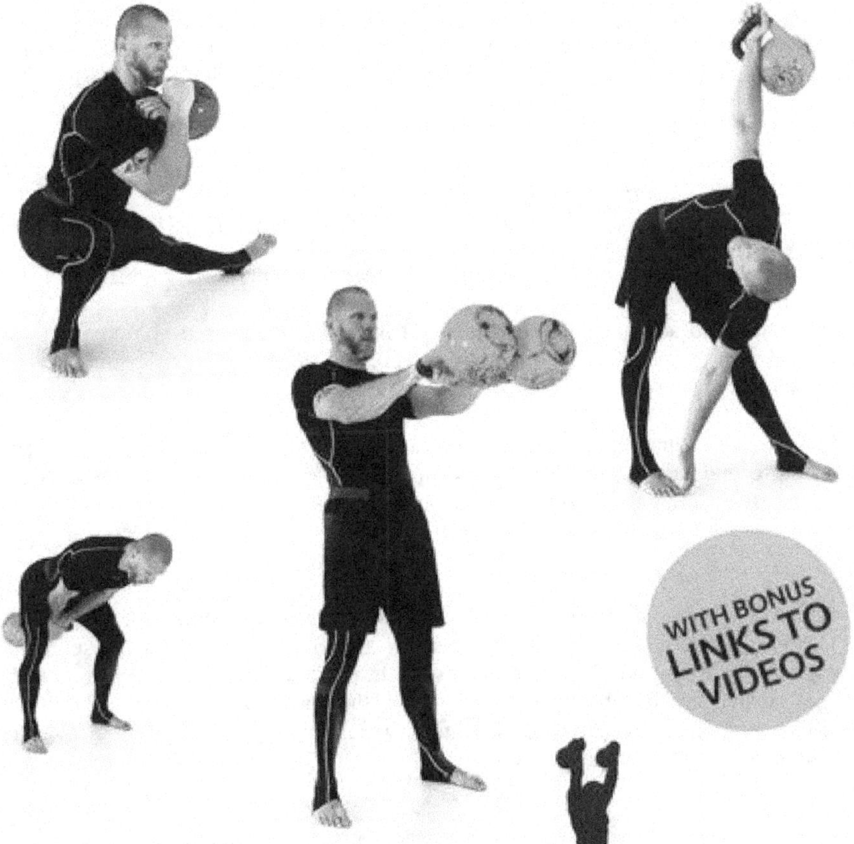

WITH BONUS **LINKS TO** VIDEOS

## By Taco Fleur from Cavemantraining

# Kettlebell Exercise Encyclopedia

Kettlebell training is a form of resistance training with the kettlebell. This book covers all kettlebell exercises with photos, descriptions, and some having step-by-step instructions. The information in this book will allow you to pick exercises and create your own kettlebell workout and/or verify that you're doing the exercises you're already doing, correctly.

The encyclopedia covers kettlebells cleans, swings, presses, lifts, snatches, squats, lunges, rows, getups, windmills, isometric exercises, isolation exercises, multi-planar exercises, combos, and more. Each subject has just enough information to keep it basic and understandable.

There are several volumes of the encyclopedia with each volume covering a set of kettlebell exercise categories. The encyclopedia is updated every 3 to 6 months with newly added exercises. If you purchased all volumes then you're entitled to download an updated digital copy from *Cavemantraining.com*, please visit go.cavemantraining.com/kbe-updates for details.

The layout and indexing of this book explained. Some exercises will have more information than others as they'll be the base for other variations. To give an example, the swing high pull contains a swing and a pull, but the swing is not explained as this would be duplicating the swing previously explained, plus, one can use different variations of the swing with the pull added.

The introduction and additional information will be repeated for each volume as it applies to all exercises and some readers might only want to purchase one particular volume that covers their subject of interest.

Compiling a resource that has each and every variation of kettlebell exercises in existence is a task that's daunting and takes time, therefore, some exercise names are listed but won't have any content, they are awaiting to be completed in the next update of the encyclopedia.

If an exercise is done with two kettlebells, and you only have two uneven kettlebells with not too much weight difference between them, let's say up to 8kg/17.6lbs max, use them. There is absolutely nothing wrong with using uneven weights, more difficult in most cases, yes, but bad, no. It does not create muscle imbalance either, in fact, the opposite, assuming you don't do anything unsound like training for months with the lighter weight on your left, and the heavier on the right side. Swap weights after a round or two.

# About the Author

My name is Taco Fleur, and I'm a Russian Girevoy Sport Institute Kettlebell Coach, IKFF Certified Kettlebell Trainer, Kettlebell Level 1 + 2 Trainer, Kettlebell Science and Application, CrossFit Level 1 Trainer, CrossFit Judges Certificate, CrossFit Programming Certificate, MMA Conditioning Level 1, MMA Fitness Level 1 + 2, Punchfit Trainer and Plyometrics Trainer Certified, with a purple belt in Brazilian Jiu-Jitsu. Author on BoxRox and featured in 4 issues of the Iron Man magazine. I have owned and set-up 3 functional kettlebell gyms in Australia and Vietnam, and lived in the Netherlands, Australia, Vietnam, and Thailand. I'm currently living in Spain.

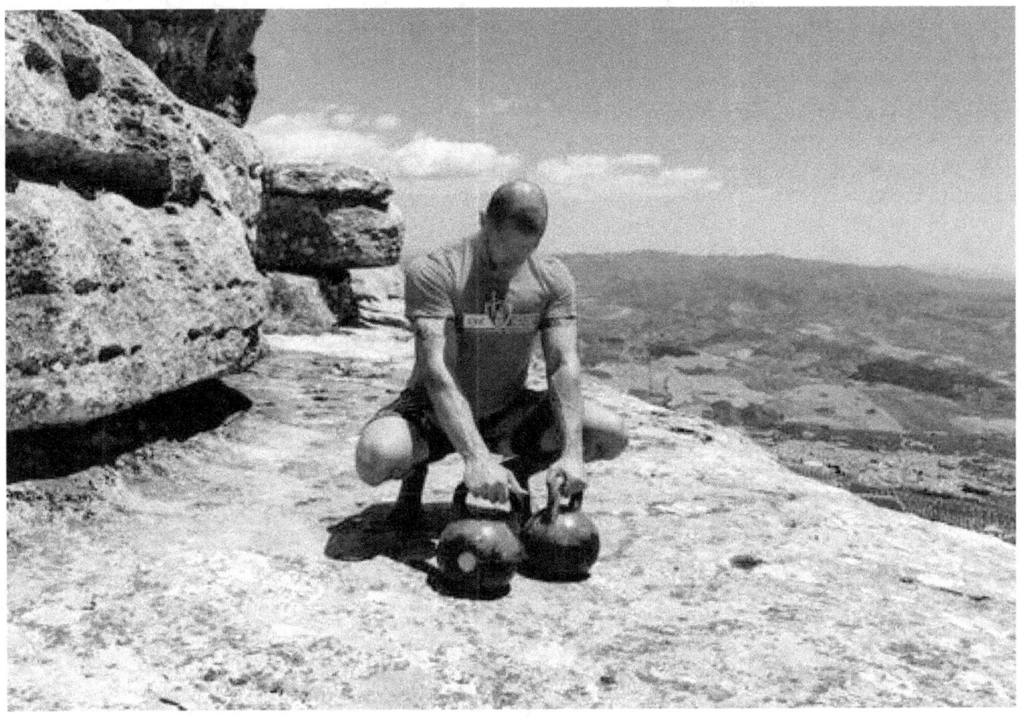

The first thing I'd like you to know about me is that I do **not** know everything, I don't pretend to know everything, and I never will. I'm on a path of life-long learning. I believe there is always something to learn from someone, no matter who they are. I've been physically active since the day I arrived on this earth in 1973. I got serious about training in 1999, touched a kettlebell for the first time in 2004, and got serious about kettlebell training in 2009. I'm here to do what I love most, and that is to share my knowledge with the world.

Some of my personal bests are 1 hour unbroken clean and jerk with a 16kg; 45 minutes unbroken clean and jerk with a 20kg; 400 burpees performed within one hour; 500 kettlebell snatches, 500 swings, and 500 double-unders completed in one session; 250 alternating dead clean and presses in one session with 20kg; 200 pull-ups in one session; 200 unbroken kettlebell swings with a 28kg; most kettlebell swings completed in one session with a 28kg (1,501); most total kettlebell swings done in 28 days with a 28kg (11,111); windmill with a 40kg kettlebell; lugged a kettlebell up a 3,479m mountain; 160kg dead lift; 100 snatches on sand with a 24kg kettlebell; 85kg Olympic Squat Snatch; 300 unbroken clean and jerk with 20kg kettlebell; 10 minute unbroken clean and jerk 80 reps with 2 x 16kg kettlebells; 532 unbroken snatches and achieved rank 2 in kettlebell sport. I mention these PBs not to boast but to demonstrate that I have a good understanding of technique and movement across different areas.

My own training and goals are geared around GPP (General Physical Preparedness) which involves kettlebell training, calisthenics, and CrossFit. I like high-volume reps but also like greasing the groove now and again. My main goals are to remains as agile as possible, remaining mobile, training in as many planes of movements as possible, and learning as many different exercise combinations and movements as possible while having fun and enjoying Brazilian Jiu-Jitsu. I'm no Arnold Schwarzenegger and never will be, but strength is not solely defined by physical appearance and huge bulging muscles.

You can read more about my training, philosophy, and other ramblings on the Cavemantraining website, www.cavemantraining.com, and on the Cavemantraining YouTube channel, bit.ly/youtube-cavemantraining, which as of this writing has over 37,000 subscribers and more than 5 million views.

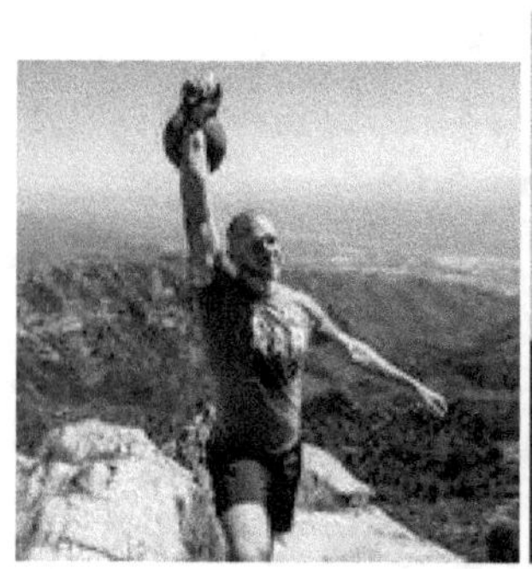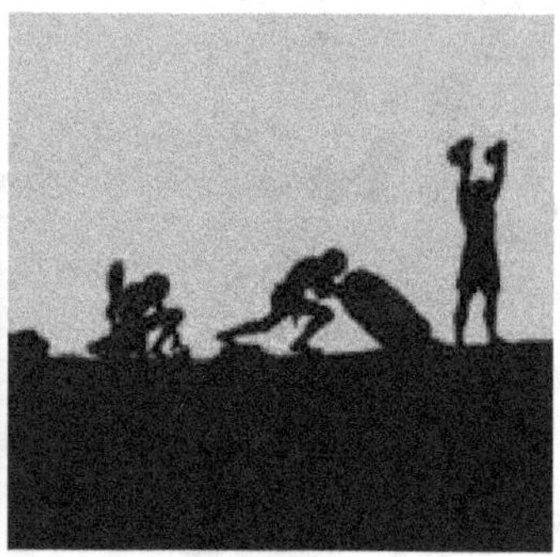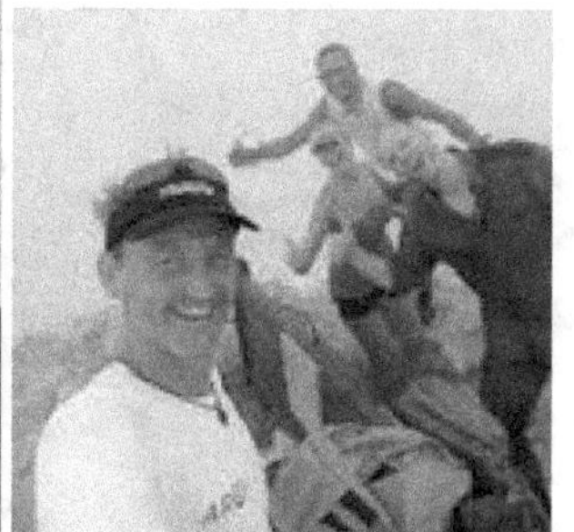

Add me: Facebook.com/taco.fleur or Facebook.com/coach.taco.fleur
Instagram: *@realcavemantraining*
Reddit: *u/cavemankettlebells*

Facebook.com/Cavemantraining or Facebook.com/Cavemantraining.Magazine
for up-to-date articles and news.

Please note that this material may not be reproduced or publicized elsewhere without the written consent of the author me@tacofleur.com.

If you bought this as a PDF/electronic copy, it is digitally signed and password protected with identifiable information.

All Cavemantraining owned images are copyrighted © Cavemantraining™

Note: Most of the <u>kettlebell stock images</u> used in this book have literally been created with blood, sweat, and tears - I'm talking about lugging kettlebells for hours up mountains, through canyons, running out of water to drink, etc. Please respect the effort that has gone into producing the photos.

Photos are available for purchase, or in some cases made available for educational purposes with appropriate credits/links in return.

# CAVEMANTRAINING

# Table of Contents

# Kettlebell Novice

If you came to this book as a kettlebell novice I can highly recommend you first check out the information on kettlebell grips and kettlebell anatomy toward the end of the book.

# Links

Please note that any links in this book are case-sensitive, this means that if you would type in go.cavemantraining.com/*KBE-VID-001* instead of go.cavemantraining.com/*kbe-vid-001* then the link will provide an error message.

# Definitions

- **Athlete**
  A person who is proficient in sports and other forms of physical exercise

- **ROM**
  Range of motion—the full and safe movement potential of a joint

- **Joint**
  A structure in the human body at which two parts of the skeleton are fitted together

- **Flexion**
  The action of bending of a limb or joint

- **Extension**
  The action of moving a limb from a bent to a straight position

- **Mobility**
  The ability to move or be moved freely and easily

- **Flexibility**
  The quality of bending easily without breaking

- **Anterior**
  Located at the front of the body

- **Posterior**
  Located at the back of the body

- **Lateral**
  Toward one side or other of the body

- **1RM**
  One repetition maximum—the maximum weight you can lift for one repetition

- **Humerus**
  The bone of the upper arm or forelimb, forming joints at the shoulder and the elbow

- **Scapulae**
  Plural for scapula (shoulder blade)

- **Spine**
  24 discs

- **Cervical**
  7 discs in the spine ranging from 1 to 7

- **Thoracic**
  12 discs in the spine ranging from 8 to 19

- **Lumbar**
  5 discs in the spine ranging from 20 to 24

- ***MMC***
  Mind muscle connection

***Ankle dorsiflexion*** is where the toes are brought closer to the shin. This decreases the angle between the dorsum of the foot and the leg. For example, when walking on the heels the ankle is described as being in dorsiflexion.

***Ankle plantar flexion*** is the opposite of dorsiflexion. Plantar flexion is the movement which decreases the angle between the sole of the foot and the back of the leg. For example, the movement when depressing a car pedal or standing on the tiptoes can be described as plantar flexion.

***Pronation*** at the forearm is a rotational movement where the hand and upper arm are turned inwards. Pronation of the foot refers to turning of the sole outwards so that weight is borne on the medial part of the foot.

***Supination*** of the forearm occurs when the forearm or palm are rotated outwards. Supination of the foot refers to turning of the sole of the foot inwards, shifting weight to the lateral edge.

***Flexion*** and ***extension*** are examples of angular motions, in which two axes of a joint are brought closer together or moved further apart. For example, elbow flexion (flex the biceps) is where you bring your hand closer toward your shoulder, and the opposite, elbow extension is where you arm moves toward being straight.

***Torque***, moment, or moment of force is rotational force. Just as a linear force is a push or a pull, a torque can be thought of as a twist to an object. In three dimensions, the torque is a pseudo-vector; for point particles, it is given by the cross product of the position vector (distance vector) and the force vector. Needless to say, torque is complex. There is always some form of torque happening during training, for the purpose of this book, I use the word to define more rotational pull being present than in other exercises, i.e. the exercise requires the body to resist more against a pulling force that wants to twist the body.

***Dead*** refers to the object not moving, not having any momentum at all before being lifted, or cleaned in our case. Dead is not to be confused with Deadlifting, which means lifting a dead weight from the ground to hanging in standing position, this can be done with a hip hinge or with a squatting movement.

# Exercise Category

When looking at kettlebell exercises they can be categorized into a parent exercise—the base exercise—and its variations, following are the most common exercises to categorize the variations by.

- Kettlebell Carry
- Kettlebell Clean
- Kettlebell Curl
- Kettlebell Getup
- Kettlebell Isometrics
- Kettlebell Kneeling
- Kettlebell Lift
- Kettlebell Lunge
- Kettlebell Press
- Kettlebell Push-up
- Kettlebell Step-up
- Kettlebell Row
- Kettlebell Snatch
- Kettlebell Squat
- Kettlebell Swing

## Kettlebell Carry

Support and move a kettlebell from one place to another. The support can be provided in the form of overhead, racked, hanging, or a mixture of aforementioned methods.

## Kettlebell Clean

A kettlebell clean is an explosive lower-body powered movement that lifts a kettlebell from a lower position to a higher position which is called racking position. The clean can be performed from the ground (dead), hanging position, or a during a ballistic movement like the swing.

Anytime a clean is performed with a swing, then that swing can be either one of the following movements, hip hinge swing, pendulum swing, or squat swing.

## Kettlebell Curl

Curl refers to the curling motion which in exercise can be performed with the elbow or knee joint, i.e. Biceps Curls or Leg Curls. Think flexion and extension of the elbow joint, or decreasing and increasing the angle of the elbow joint. When it comes to kettlebell training the common curling exercise used is the biceps curl, although technically speaking the leg curl could be performed laying down and the foot through the window of the kettlebell.

## Kettlebell Get-up

To get up into a fully erect position any way possible from laying flat on the floor. This can be done with 1 or 2 kettlebells positioned overhead or racked.

## Kettlebell Isometrics

Isometric relates to muscular action in which tension is developed without contraction of the muscle. There is no movement, action, or change, also known as static. A good example of an isometric exercise is the plank or iron cross. Isometrics can also be mixed with dynamic exercise, for example, a squat with frontal hold.

## Kettlebell Kneeling

To kneel means to be in or assume a position in which the body is supported by a knee or the knees. You can perform movements into kneeling positions like surrenders or you can perform exercises in which you remain in kneeling position like kneeling hip thrusts.

## Kettlebell Lift

To lift something means to raise to a higher position or level. In effect, almost all kettlebell exercises could be thought of like a lift, i.e. snatch, press, clean, swing, etc. However, we're going to classify a lift as a movement in which the kettlebell is brought from a low to a higher position via a slow movement. We're excluding explosive movements as they have their own classifications, i.e. press, snatch, clean, and swing.

## Kettlebell Lunge

To define the lunge a few assumptions will be made. The dictionary defines the word as making a sudden forward thrust with part of the body, in our context that part of the body would be the leg. A lunge is also the basic attacking move in fencing, which is very similar to the lunge exercise as we know it. The lunge as we know it not only moves forward but all different directions, back (reverse), side, etc. The difference between the lunge used in fencing and exercise is that the back knee usually bends and gently taps the floor to set a standard for depth.

## Kettlebell Press

The press and push movement are very similar when you look at the arms, they're always extending, whether overhead or above the chest (laying down), however, there is a clear difference between the two. With the press, you exert physical force on the kettlebell to move it away from you rather than to move yourself away from it (push).

## Kettlebell Push-up

Similar to the press, you exert physical force on the kettlebell, but in this case, it's in order to move yourself away from it. A push-up done on the floor would be pushing yourself away from the floor. If you take the same push-up position and turn it around—laying flat—and perform the same movement it becomes as press as you're moving the object away from yourself.

## Kettlebell Step-up

A step-up is performed by placing one foot onto a higher plateau and pushing yourself up by exerting force and extending the working leg. You can perform step-ups on box jumps, stairs, or other suitable objects.

## Kettlebell Row

When looking at the movement in boat rowing it's always a pull and push off the oar. In the context of kettlebell training, a row is always a pull as gravity replaces the push. A row has to be performed in such a way that you're acting directly against gravity. The focus of the kettlebell row are the posterior muscles of the upper back.

## Kettlebell Snatch

A snatch is a movement in which the kettlebell rapidly raised from a lower position—always below the hips—to above the head in one continuous smooth explosive movement. An example of a few common start positions are dead, hanging, and swinging.

## Kettlebell Squat

The squat is a movement in which three joints flex, namely the ankle, knee, and hip joints. During the movement, the objective is to get the hips as low to the ground as possible while keeping the shoulders as high as possible. The squat can be performed in with the kettlebell(s) overhead, racked, or dead, however, when dead, it will be moved to the category of a lift.

## Kettlebell Swing

A swing takes place when an object moves back and forth or from side to side while suspended. The swing is the foundation for many other exercises, such as the clean and snatch. The swing can be actioned as a pull or pendulum. The most common variation outside of the sport world is the pulling version whereas in the sport world it's the opposite and the pendulum is common.

# List by Name

The following index is all kettlebell exercises by name. Note that not all variations are included in this book. The first column is the name, the second column is the variation, combine the two together and you have the full name, for example, *Carry Racked* would become *Racked Carry*. If it's single-arm and single kettlebell then it can be the left or right side and one arm is not working. If it's double-hand and single kettlebell then both hands are holding on to the kettlebell. If it's double-hand and double kettlebell then both sides have a kettlebell. If the hand is marked as alternating then that's a variation where the kettlebell goes from one side to the other.

| **Name** | Variation | Hand | Kettlebell |
|---|---|---|---|
| **Carry** | Racked | Single | Single |
| **Carry** | Racked | Double | Double |
| **Carry** | Goblet | Double | Single |
| **Carry** | Overhead | Single | Single |
| **Carry** | Overhead | Double | Double |
| **Carry** | Suitcase | Single | Single |
| **Carry** | Suitcase | Double | Double |
| **Carry** | Waiter | Single | Single |
| **Carry** | Waiter | Double | Double |
| **Clean** | Assisted Dead | Single | Single |
| **Clean** | Assisted Hang | Single | Single |
| **Clean** | Assisted Swing | Single | Single |
| **Clean** | Assisted Dead Swing | Single | Single |
| **Clean** | Dead | Single | Single |
| **Clean** | Dead | Alternating | Single |
| **Clean** | Dead | Double | Double |
| **Clean** | Hang | Single | Single |
| **Clean** | Hang | Alternating | Single |
| **Clean** | Hang | Double | Double |
| **Clean** | Gorilla | Double | Double |
| **Clean** | Swing | Single | Single |
| **Clean** | Swing | Alternating | Single |
| **Clean** | Swing | Double | Single |
| **Clean** | Swing | Double | Double |
| **Clean** | Pendulum | Single | Single |
| **Clean** | Pendulum | Alternating | Single |

| Name | Variation | Hand | Kettlebell |
| --- | --- | --- | --- |
| **Clean** | Pendulum | Double | Double |
| **Clean** | Half Circular | Single | Single |
| **Clean** | Circular | Single | Single |
| **Clean** | Goblet | Double | Single |
| **Clean** | Horn | Double | Single |
| **Clean** | Bottoms-up Horn | Double | Single |
| **Clean** | Suitcase | Single | Single |
| **Clean** | Suitcase | Double | Double |
| **Clean** | Suitcase | Alternating | Double |
| **Clean** | Suitcase Hang | Single | Single |
| **Clean** | Suitcase Hang | Double | Double |
| **Clean** | Suitcase Hang | Alternating | Double |
| **Clean** | Lawnmower | Single | Single |
| **Clean** | Lawnmower | Double | Double |
| **Clean** | Lawnmower | Double | Single |
| **Curl** | Conventional | Single | Single |
| **Curl** | Conventional | Double | Single |
| **Curl** | Conventional | Double | Double |
| **Curl** | Conventional | Alternating | Double |
| **Curl** | Hammer | Single | Single |
| **Curl** | Hammer | Double | Single |
| **Curl** | Hammer | Double | Double |
| **Curl** | Squat Dead | Single | Single |
| **Curl** | Squat Dead | Double | Double |
| **Curl** | Gorilla | Single | Single |
| **Curl** | Gorilla | Alternating | Double |
| **Curl** | Gorilla | Double | Double |
| **Curl** | Bent Side | Single | Single |
| **Getup** | Turkish Lunge | Single | Single |
| **Getup** | Turkish Squat | Single | Single |
| **Getup** | Racked | Double | Double |
| **Getup** | Shin Box Racked | Single | Single |
| **Getup** | Shin Box Racked | Double | Double |
| **Getup** | Shin Box Overhead | Single | Single |

| Name | Variation | Hand | Kettlebell |
|---|---|---|---|
| **Getup** | Shin Box Overhead | Double | Double |
| **Isometrics** | Crucifix | Double | Double |
| **Isometrics** | Frontal Hold | Double | Single |
| **Isometrics** | L-sit | Double | Double |
| **Isometrics** | Spartan Side Plank | Single | Single |
| **Lift** | Racked Deadlift | Double | Double |
| **Lift** | Hang Squat/Hip Hinge | Single | Single |
| **Lift** | Hang Squat/Hip Hinge | Double | Single |
| **Lift** | Hang Squat/Hip Hinge | Double | Double |
| **Lift** | Dead Squat/Hip Hinge | Single | Single |
| **Lift** | Dead Squat/Hip Hinge | Alternating | Single |
| **Lift** | Dead Squat/Hip Hinge | Double | Single |
| **Lift** | Dead Squat/Hip Hinge | Double | Double |
| **Lift** | Suitcase | Single | Single |
| **Lift** | Suitcase | Alternating | Double |
| **Lift** | Suitcase | Double | Double |
| **Lift** | Sumo Dead Squat/Hip Hinge | Single | Single |
| **Lift** | Sumo Dead Squat/Hip Hinge | Double | Single |
| **Lift** | Sumo Dead Squat/Hip Hinge | Alternating | Single |
| **Lift** | Sumo Dead Squat/Hip Hinge | Double | Double |
| **Lift** | Dead Stiff-legged | Single | Single |
| **Lift** | Dead Stiff-legged | Double | Double |
| **Lift** | Dead Stiff-legged | Alternating | Double |
| **Lunge** | Forward/Reverse Racked | Single | Single |
| **Lunge** | Forward/Reverse Racked | Double | Single |
| **Lunge** | Forward/Reverse Racked | Double | Double |
| **Lunge** | Forward/Reverse Overhead | Single | Single |
| **Lunge** | Forward/Reverse Overhead | Double | Double |
| **Lunge** | Curtsy Racked | Single | Single |
| **Lunge** | Curtsy Racked | Double | Single |
| **Lunge** | Curtsy Racked | Double | Double |
| **Lunge** | Curtsy Overhead | Single | Single |
| **Lunge** | Curtsy Overhead | Double | Double |
| **Press** | Front/Hybrid/Side | Single | Single |

| Name | Variation | Hand | Kettlebell |
| --- | --- | --- | --- |
| **Press** | Front/Hybrid/Side | Alternating | Double |
| **Press** | Front/Hybrid/Side | Double | Double |
| **Press** | Rear | Single | Single |
| **Press** | Seesaw | Double | Double |
| **Press** | Bent Side | Single | Single |
| **Press** | Push | Single | Single |
| **Press** | Push | Double | Double |
| **Press** | Sots | Single | Single |
| **Press** | Sots | Alternating | Double |
| **Press** | Sots | Double | Double |
| **Press** | Seated | Single | Single |
| **Press** | Seated | Alternating | Double |
| **Press** | Seated | Double | Double |
| **Press** | Chest | Single | Single |
| **Press** | Chest | Alternating | Double |
| **Press** | Chest | Double | Double |
| **Press** | Spiral | Single | Single |
| **Row** | Bent-over Lunge (Diff. angles) | Single | Single |
| **Row** | Bent-over (Diff. angles) | Single | Single |
| **Row** | Bent-over (Diff. angles) | Alternating | Double |
| **Row** | Bent-over (Diff. angles) | Double | Double |
| **Row** | Renegade | Double | Double |
| **Snatch** | Half Hip Hinge/Squat/Pendulum | Single | Single |
| **Snatch** | Half Hip Hinge/Squat/Pendulum | Alternating | Single |
| **Snatch** | Half Hip Hinge/Squat/Pendulum | Double | Double |
| **Snatch** | Full Hip Hinge/Squat/Pendulum | Single | Single |
| **Snatch** | Full Hip Hinge/Squat/Pendulum | Alternating | Single |
| **Snatch** | Full Hip Hinge/Squat/Pendulum | Double | Double |
| **Snatch** | Dead Half | Single | Single |
| **Snatch** | Dead Half | Alternating | Single |
| **Snatch** | Dead Half | Double | Double |
| **Snatch** | Dead Full | Single | Single |
| **Snatch** | Dead Full | Alternating | Single |
| **Snatch** | Dead Full | Double | Double |

| Name | Variation | Hand | Kettlebell |
| --- | --- | --- | --- |
| **Squat** | Racked | Single | Single |
| **Squat** | Racked | Double | Single |
| **Squat** | Racked | Double | Double |
| **Squat** | Deck | Double | Single |
| **Squat** | Pistol | Double | Single |
| **Squat** | Goblet | Double | Single |
| **Squat** | Overhead | Single | Single |
| **Squat** | Overhead | Double | Double |
| **Squat** | Back | Single | Single |
| **Squat** | Back | Double | Double |
| **Squat** | Cossack Racked | Single | Single |
| **Squat** | Cossack Racked | Double | Double |
| **Squat** | Cossack Overhead | Single | Single |
| **Squat** | Cossack Overhead | Double | Double |
| **Squat** | Thruster | Single | Single |
| **Squat** | Thruster | Double | Double |
| **Squat** | Hindu Racked | Single | Single |
| **Squat** | Hindu Racked | Double | Double |
| **Squat** | Hindu Overhead | Single | Single |
| **Squat** | Hindu Overhead | Double | Double |
| **Swing** | Hip Hinge/Squat/Pendulum | Single | Single |
| **Swing** | Hip Hinge/Squat/Pendulum | Alternating | Single |
| **Swing** | Hip Hinge/Squat/Pendulum | Double | Double |
| **Swing** | American | Double | Single |
| **Swing** | Atlas | Single | Single |
| **Swing** | Atlas | Double | Single |
| **Swing** | Short Lever | Double | Single |
| **Swing** | Gorilla | Single | Single |
| **Swing** | Gorilla | Double | Single |
| **Swing** | Gorilla | Double | Double |
| **Swing** | Power | Double | Single |
| **Jerk** | Conventional | Single | Single |
| **Jerk** | Conventional | Double | Double |
| **Jerk** | Split | Single | Single |

| **Name** Variation | Hand | Kettlebell |
| --- | --- | --- |
| **Jerk** Split | Double | Double |
| **Jerk** Squat | Single | Single |
| **Jerk** Squat | Double | Double |

The objective was to keep the list brief as there are plenty more variations than those listed. Just by changing up the grip on a clean you have a variation, for example, a dead clean with a waiters grip would become a waiters clean, a swing clean with an open palm would become an open palm swing clean, and so on. I purposely chosen not to do that with the above list. There is a list online which has more variation if you're interested.

http://bit.ly/kettlebell-exercise-list

# List With Goal

The following list are all kettlebell exercises listed with their goal. The goals are generalized as the most common goals used for those exercises, but not meaning that's all they're good for. It should also be noted that most goals can change through programming. With the goals being:

- Muscular strength
- Cardiovascular endurance
  - Aerobic
  - Anaerobic
- Flexibility
- Balance
- Stability
- Mobility
- Agility
- Power
- Speed
- Cardiovascular endurance
- Muscular endurance
- Core

## Cardiovascular Endurance

Cardiovascular endurance is how efficiently your heart, blood vessels, and lungs supply oxygen-rich blood to working muscles during physical activity for a prolonged period of time, usually for more than 90 seconds. You improve your cardiovascular endurance when you improve the capacity of the muscles to extract oxygen from the bloodstream to produce energy. Your cardiovascular endurance is improved when you can maintain an increased heart rate and breathing rate for a longer period of time than you were previously capable.

## Balance

Balance is your ability to maintain an even distribution of weight enabling you to remain upright and steady during movement or static position.

## Stability

Although often confused, stability is not the same as balance. Stability is the ability to prevent something from moving, it requires strength and a good mind-muscle connection.

## Agility

Agility is the ability to move quickly and easily.

## Power

Power is a combination of speed and strength.

## Speed

Speed is very similar to power with the biggest difference being that the weight used is much lighter so to be able to maintain high-speed contractions with low resistance.

## Muscular Endurance

Muscular endurance is a particular muscle's ability to continuously contract against a given resistance. A good example of this is the iron cross exercise in which your whole body is engaged and contracted, the longer you're able to stay in this position the greater your muscular endurance is. In other words, it defines how fatigue-resistant particular muscles are.

## Muscular Strength

Muscular strength is the ability to perform one repetition at your maximal intensity. In other words, the amount of force particular muscles can produce in one, all-out effort.

## Flexibility

The ability of a muscle or muscle groups to lengthen passively through a range of motion.

## Mobility

Mobility is a combination of qualities that make it easy to come in and out of maximum range of any given muscle. Some qualities but not limited to are stability, strength, mind-muscle connection, etc.

## Core

The muscles that attach to the spine and pelvis are referred to as the core muscles. Just about any exercise done while standing places a demand on the core muscles, but there are those that place and increased demand and those will be categorized here.

| Name | Variation | Goal |
|---|---|---|
| **Carry** | Racked/Goblet | Muscular endurance, muscular strength, core |
| **Carry** | Overhead | Muscular endurance, muscular strength, core, stability, flexibility |
| **Carry** | Suitcase | Muscular endurance, muscular strength, core, stability |
| **Clean** | Assisted | Technique, drilling |
| **Clean** | Dead/Hang | Muscular strength, cardiovascular endurance, flexibility, power, muscular endurance, core |
| **Clean** | Gorilla | Muscular strength, cardiovascular endurance (anaerobic), power, core |
| **Clean** | Swing | Muscular strength, cardiovascular endurance (aerobic/anaerobic), core |
| **Clean** | Pendulum | Cardiovascular endurance (aerobic), muscular endurance, core |
| **Clean** | Suitcase/Suitcase Hang | Muscular strength, cardiovascular endurance, flexibility, power, muscular endurance, core |
| **Curl** | Conventional/Hammer | Muscular strength |
| **Curl** | Squat Dead/Gorilla/Bent Side | Muscular strength, flexibility |
| **Getup** | Turkish Lunge/Turkish Squat/Racked/Shin Box Racked/Shin Box Overhead | Muscular strength, muscular endurance, flexibility, mobility, stability, core |
| **Isometrics** | Crucifix/Frontal Hold/L-sit/Spartan Side Plank | Muscular strength, muscular endurance, stability, core |
| **Lift** | All variations | Muscular strength, flexibility, core |
| **Lunge** | Forward Racked | Muscular strength, flexibility, stability, core, explosive strength |
| **Lunge** | Reverse Racked | Muscular strength, flexibility, stability, core |
| **Lunge** | Curtsy Racked/Curtsy Overhead | Muscular strength, muscular endurance, flexibility, mobility, stability, core |
| **Press** | Front/Hybrid/Side | Muscular strength, flexibility, core |
| **Press** | Rear | Muscular strength, flexibility, mobility, core |
| **Press** | Seesaw | Muscular strength, muscular |

| Name | Variation | Goal |
| --- | --- | --- |
| | | endurance, flexibility, mobility, core |
| **Press** | Bent Side | Muscular strength, flexibility, mobility, core |
| **Press** | Push | Muscular strength, cardiovascular endurance, flexibility, power, core |
| **Press** | Sots | Muscular strength, muscular endurance, flexibility, mobility, stability, core |
| **Press** | Seated | Muscular strength, muscular endurance, flexibility |
| **Press** | Chest | Muscular strength |
| **Press** | Spiral | Muscular strength, muscular endurance, flexibility, mobility, stability, core |
| **Row** | Bent-over Lunge (Diff. angles) | Muscular strength, muscular endurance, flexibility, stability |
| **Row** | Bent-over (Diff. angles)/Renegade | Muscular strength, muscular endurance, flexibility, stability, core |
| **Snatch** | Half Hip Hinge/Squat | Power, muscular strength, muscular endurance, flexibility, cardiovascular endurance (aerobic/anaerobic), core |
| **Snatch** | Half Pendulum | Muscular endurance, cardiovascular endurance (aerobic), core |
| **Snatch** | Dead Half/Dead Full | Explosive strength, power, flexibility, cardiovascular endurance (anaerobic), muscular strength, core |
| **Squat** | Racked/Goblet/Overhead/Back | Muscular strength, muscular endurance, flexibility, core |
| **Squat** | Deck | Mobility, flexibility |
| **Squat** | Pistol | Muscular strength, muscular endurance, flexibility, core, stability, balance |
| **Squat** | Thruster | Muscular strength, power, muscular endurance, cardiovascular endurance (anaerobic), flexibility |
| **Squat** | Cossack Overhead/Cossack Racked/Hindu Racked/Hindu Overhead | Muscular strength, muscular endurance, flexibility, stability, mobility, core |
| **Swing** | Hip Hinge/Squat/Power | Muscular strength, power, cardiovascular endurance (aerobic/anaerobic), flexibility, core |

| Name | Variation | Goal |
| --- | --- | --- |
| **Swing** | Pendulum | Cardiovascular endurance (aerobic), core |
| **Swing** | American | Muscular strength, cardiovascular endurance (aerobic/anaerobic), flexibility, core |
| **Swing** | Atlas/Gorilla | Muscular strength, cardiovascular endurance, flexibility, core |
| **Jerk** | Conventional/Split/Squat | Muscular strength, cardiovascular endurance (aerobic/anaerobic), flexibility, core |

# Common Kettlebell References

Following are common kettlebell references used within many other exercises and thus important to list upfront so that it's easy to understand when referenced to later.

# Hyperextension

## What is Hip (Hyper)extension?

Our definition for hyperextension is most likely different from other writings you might have encountered. Haven written over 10 books and courses it has become obvious that the following definition of hyperextension works better for clarity and avoiding addition descriptions. Caveat: The hyperextension definition that follows should only be considered under the context of Cavemantraining material.

Hip flexion is where you pull the top of the pelvis down towards the ground, and extension is the opposite. Hip hyperextension is not something everyone can do right away, you need flexibility at the front, something you'll need to work on over a duration of time.

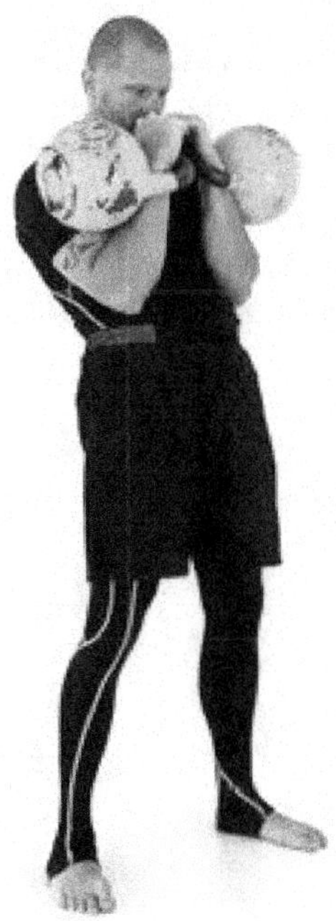

In a neutral position you'd be in extension, going further back, i.e. pulling the pelvis further back, is called hip hyperextension. But most people associate 'injury' with the word hyperextension, and its definition is:

> Hyperextension is an excessive joint movement in which the angle formed by the bones of a particular joint is opened, or straightened, beyond its normal, healthy, range of motion.

Hyper means: over; beyond; above.

Hyperextension without flexibility is indeed a cause for injury and hyperextension in joints that are not made to hyperextend is also cause for injury. Hyperextension with proper flexibility and progression is something everyone should strive for. Joints that can be hyperextended through a proper progression are:

- Hips
- Spine (back/neck)

You create hip extension by squeezing the gluteus maximus and letting the top of the femur come slightly forward, i.e. normally positioned above the ankles, now coming forward towards the toes. This action tilts the pelvis backward. On top of the pelvis is the spine, this follows along naturally—resembling back hyperextension—if you keep it positioned neutrally.

The second step is to crunch, bring the shoulders and head forward, this is done via thoracic flexion, the same action you make when performing crunches on the ground.

Racking should not be confused with back hyperextension, although back hyperextensions are also something one should be doing, and is completely safe with proper progression, it is however, not a safe nor an efficient position to rest in with heavy weights. Back hyperextension is actually the complete opposite of what a good racking position is. A good racking position is with thoracic flexion (think crunching), hip hyperextension, with knee extension, and slight ankle dorsiflexion.

# Hike Back

The hike back is one of the most common movements used for starting swings, snatches, cleans, or anything that requires the bell to come from the ground and then out and up. The most common movement to perform this with is the hip hinge but a squat can also be used. The most important safety points are:

- Neutral spine

- Kettlebells come through just under or around knee height

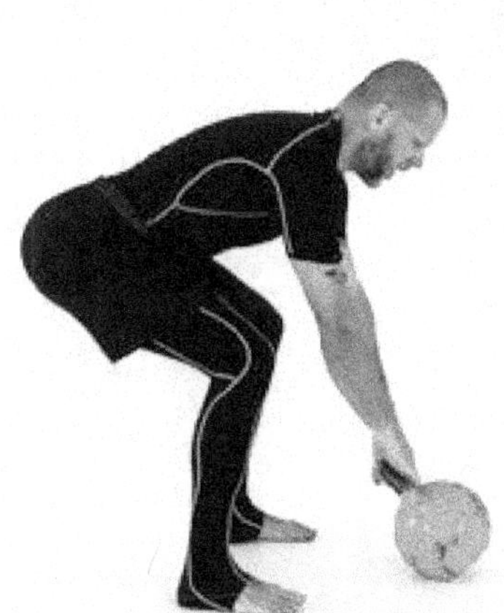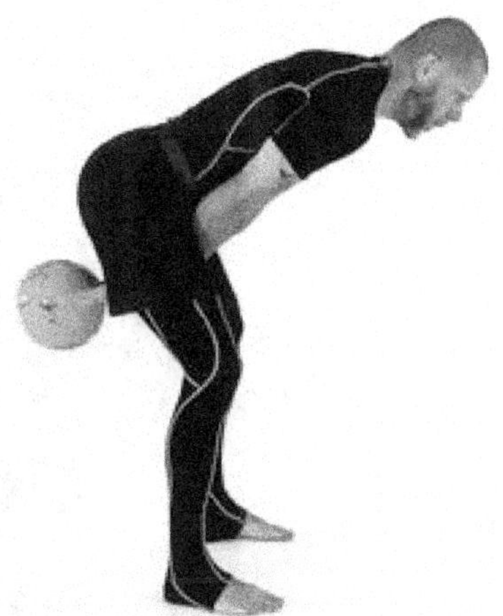

The pull should be controlled and not violent. The pull should bring the arms into a gentle connection with the body as demonstrated in the second photo above. The pull can only be safe and natural when there is enough space between you and the kettlebell, without sufficient space, it will turn into a push between the legs rather than a pull. The space required is different from person to person but as long as the same position as demonstrated in the first photo is achieved it will be safe.

**Kettlebells come through just under or around knee height.**

This will all vary depending on body composition but the main thing to keep in mind is to keep the shoulders above the hips with a neutral spine. Direct the weights to the back rather than low to the ground, low to the ground would mean a pull up is required, whereas far back would give you momentum from the kettlebells using gravity. This is not to say that performing this with a pull is bad, it can be good if its what your goal requires, but in general this movement is performed to take advantage of momentum.

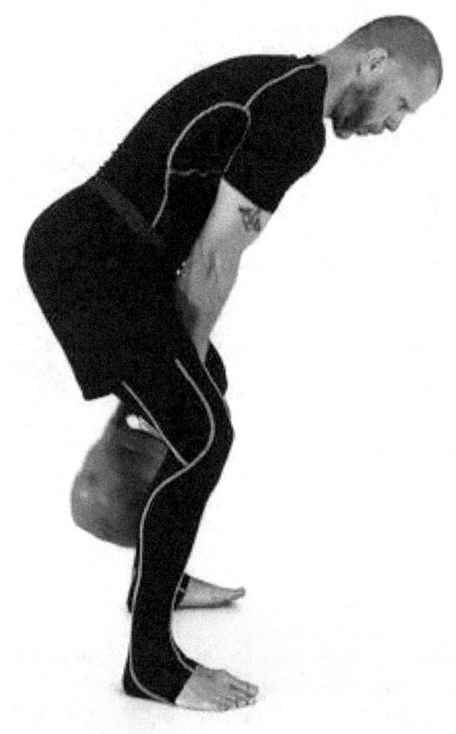

The hike back can be performed with one or two kettlebells, and with one or two arms. When using two kettlebells you will need to use a wider stance but at the same time making sure the knees don't buckle out.

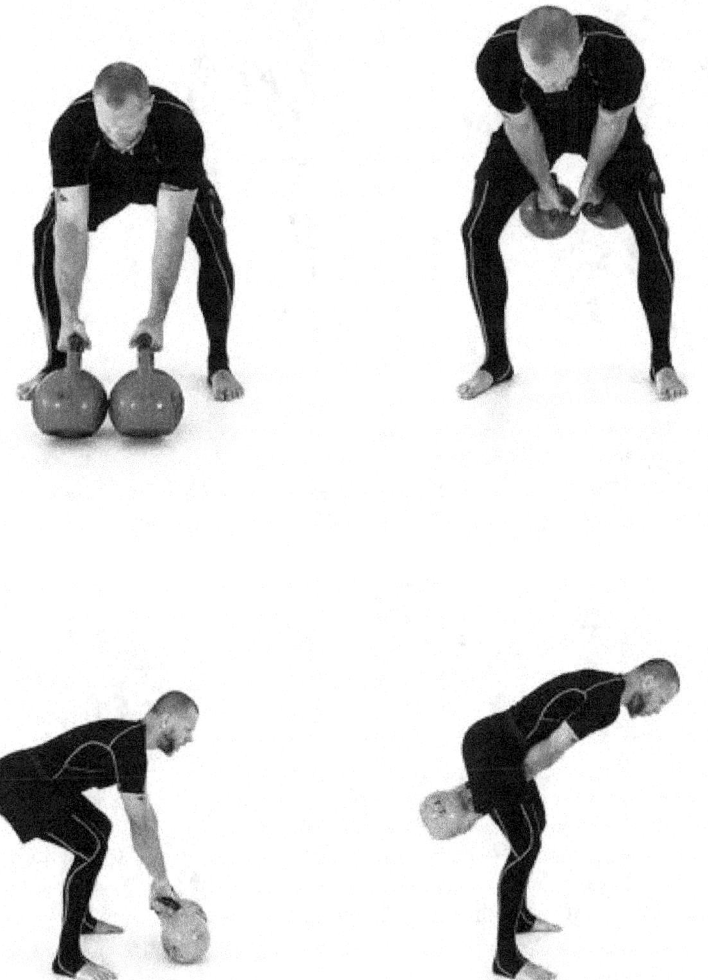

Always create some tension between you and the weight before pulling. See the first photo.

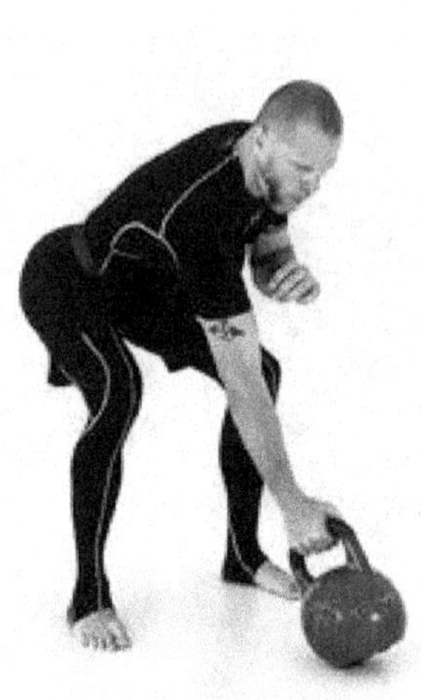 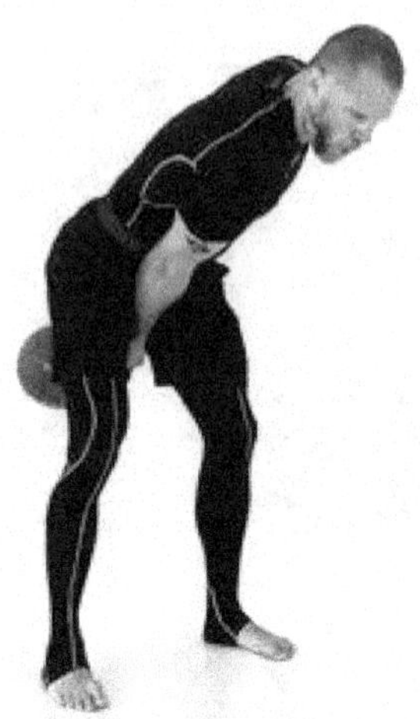

The hike back is commonly part of or used to transition into another exercise, but it can just as well be used as an exercise on its own, and I personally use it to break down the kettlebell swing and perfect the position into which the backswing should end. This looks as following.

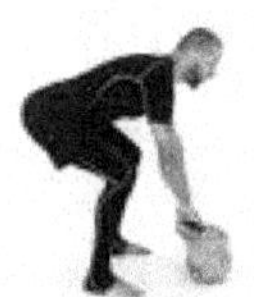 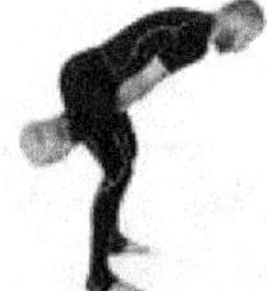 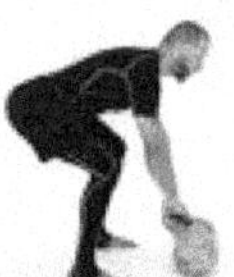 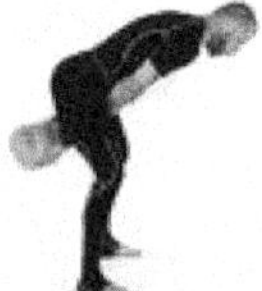 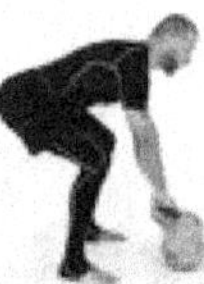

Apart from it teaching the athlete what the end of the backswing should feel like, it also engrains the position for the first part of starting a swing. The main areas worked here are the posterior chain muscles and the quadriceps. For the pull, all muscles responsible for shoulder extension are used. There is minimal movement when it comes to hip or knee extension, hence, this is mostly isometric apart from the pull.

# Counterbalance

Looking at the dictionary for the word *counterbalance*:

- a weight that balances another weight.

- a factor having the opposite effect to that of another and so preventing it from exercising a disproportionate influence.

The following photos are a great example of good counterbalance during the drop from the rack. As the weights fall forward the upper body comes back and away from the weights which creates an even counterbalance to prevent disproportionate load on the lower back.

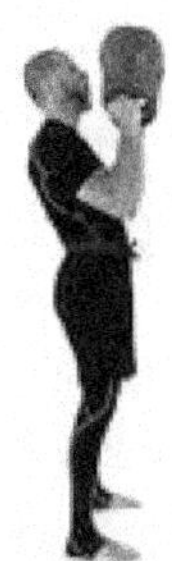 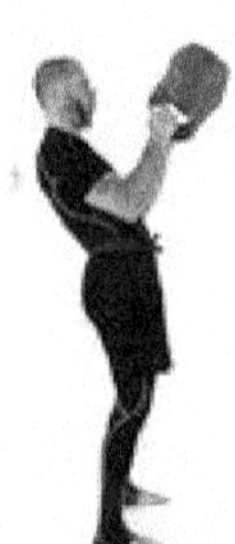 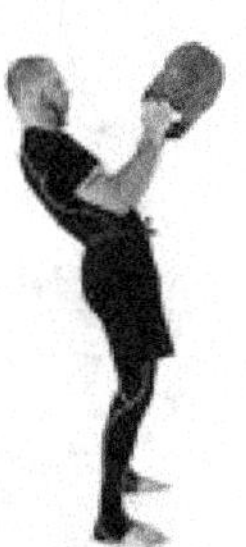 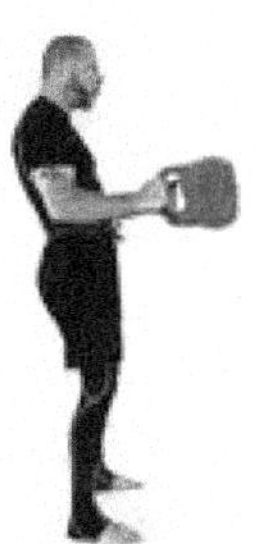

The amount of counterbalance required increases with the amount of weight used, the heavier the weight the more one needs to work on counterbalancing during movements. There are several areas through which counterbalance can be created:

- Ankles (plantar flexion)
- Knees (flexion)
- Hips (hyperextension)
- Thoracic spine (hyperextension)

# Drop

Whether you're dropping the weight from racking or overhead, you should never follow the kettlebell. What this means is, as soon as you initiate the drop, don't bend at the hips too, if you're bending at the hips the moment the weight drops (comes forward) then you're compromising your lower back, you're putting unnecessary pressure/stress on it. With the drop from rack you want to be in extension or even hyperextension, at the point the bell is around/below the hip area which all depends on whether the arm is straight or not, if it's not, don't come out of extension yet. The same applies to the full drop from overhead, however, due to the kettlebell being further away from the body, the arm will be extended sooner, hence, the follow-through happens sooner than with the drop from the rack.

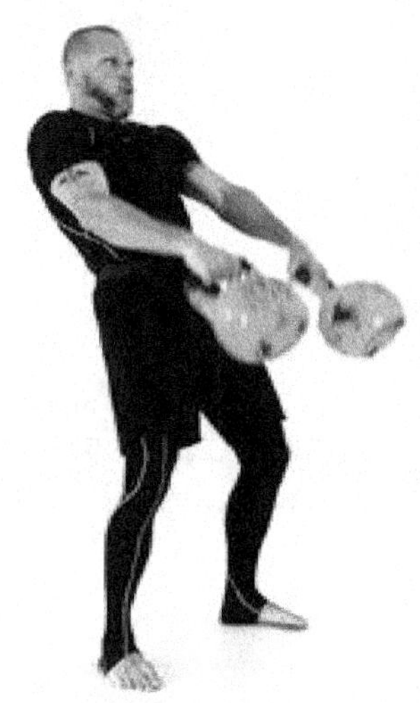

More information on this topic can be found under the clean and swing.

A good example of the drop can be seen in slow-motion in this video go.cavemantraining.com/kbe-vid-001

# Rack/Racking

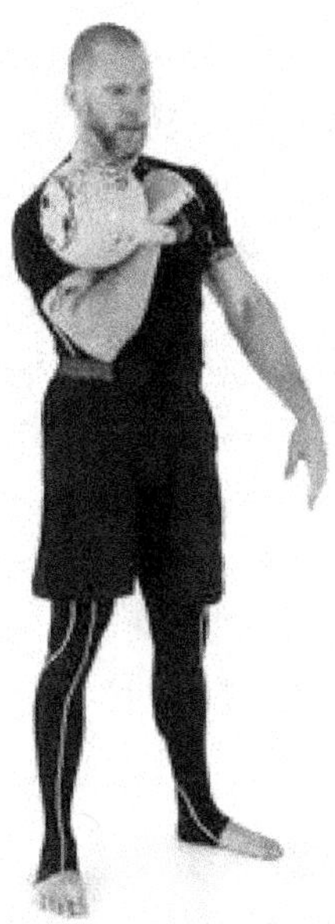

Dot points:

- Kettlebell racking happens after you clean a kettlebell

- The rack can be a resting or transitional position

- A bad racking position can burn out the shoulders or affect the forearm

- With a transitional rack your elbow should be tucked/pulled into your obliques/ribs

- Use your latissimus dorsi to pull the elbow/arm in

- Rest the bell on the biceps and forearm

- A little bit of space at the bottom of the elbow is ok for a transitional rack

- Place the elbow on the ilium to transfer power for jerking or push pressing

- For resting you want to rest the elbow on the ilium

- During sport/endurance/high volume reps you want to use a good rack to be able to rest with the bell up

- A disconnected arm means shoulder flexion which means additional and unnecessary work

- Let the weight rest on your skeletal system and not your muscular system

- Although it might look like it's bad for the lumbar there is actually no movement in the lumbar

- All range is created through hip hyperextension and extension plus flexion in the thoracic

- A good rack requires flexibility in the hips and thoracic

- Squeeze the gluteus maximus to pull the top of the pelvis back

- Let the top of the femur come slightly forward

- Getting better range in the hip flexors takes time

- Hip hyperextension and crunch

- A rounded back is not a problem because we're not pressing

- You want to rack with just enough contraction to obtain a good posture

- The weight naturally wants to fall away from the body which requires work to pull in

- Make space to let the weight rest on/above the legs

- A cradle rack is an option for females with larger breasts

- The rack is a position you need to learn properly

# Kettlebell Exercises

A kettlebell exercise, in effect, is a bodyweight exercise to which resistance is added in the form of a kettlebell. An exercise has variations. Several exercises strung together become a combo (combination). In this encyclopedia of kettlebell exercises I will cover the purest form of an exercise, variations, and some combinations as a bonus.

# Kettlebell Squat

The squat is a super important exercise for overall well-being and an exercise I will devote some time to learning with just bodyweight. Although a great exercise, an exercise that should be done correctly or many issues can arise. You need a good range of ankle dorsiflexion, if you do not have that then you'll most likely be leaning forward to compensate or fall backward when going deep. The squat brings you many other benefits like calf, quad, gluteals, and back strength, most people don't look at the squat as a back exercise when done with just **bodyweight**, but once you understand how much back work is required to keep those shoulders up and the spine neutrally aligned, then you'll understand how good the squat is for your back.

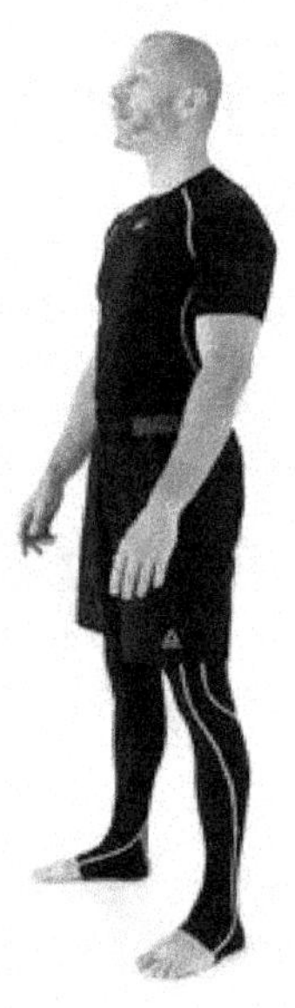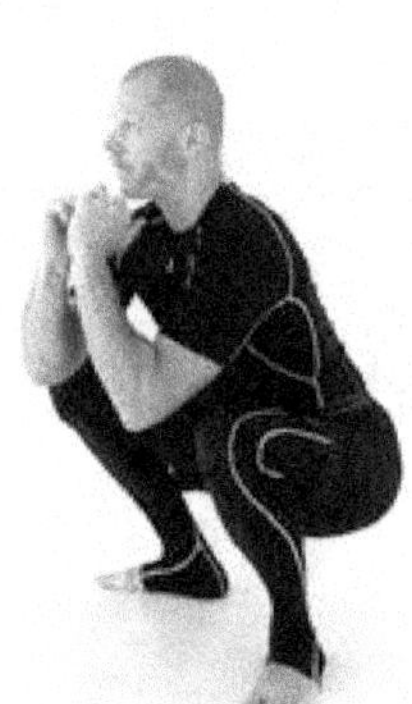

**To perform:**

- Stand in a wider than neutral stance

- The feet should be pointing slightly out at an angle

- Keep the hands in front of your chest or let them hang but do not use them for balancing

- Press the heels into the ground to create tension in the hamstrings

- Press the balls of the feet into the ground for a good grounding

- Slightly pull the top of the feet away from each other through hip lateral rotation but without actually moving the feet (create tension)

- Contract the quadriceps

- Keep looking ahead throughout the movement

- Break at all three joints at the same time

- Slowly release as little tension as is required to create flexion (ankle = dorsiflexion)

- Maintain balance and even weight distribution by adjusting how much the knees come forward and the hips back

- The hips keep traveling down till maximum range is achieved

- The shoulders follow the hips which means that the shoulders do not move down unless the hips do

- The back should stay neutrally aligned or slightly hyperextended but not rounded

- There should **always** be good alignment between all joints which is dictated by you pulling the knees laterally out to maintain this alignment

- At maximum depth do not release tension

- Come back up the same way you came down

**Maximum range** is your maximum range that's achieved safely and with good technique, this might mean only 50% of someone else's full range, but that doesn't matter, just focus on safety and technique.

The squat is a strength exercise but at the same time good for mobility and flexibility. You'll receive strength from resistance and time under tension, the deeper you go the longer you're under tension and the more strength is required. On that note, when the instructions ask for tension through contraction or pressing, that tension remains unless specified otherwise.

Alignment between the ankles, knees, and hips means that if you would draw a line from the top to the bottom all joints would be within that line. For example, a line connecting one ankle and hip joint but not the knee means that the knee is either buckled in or too far out, either one will provide stress on the knee joint.

# SQUAT ALIGNMENT

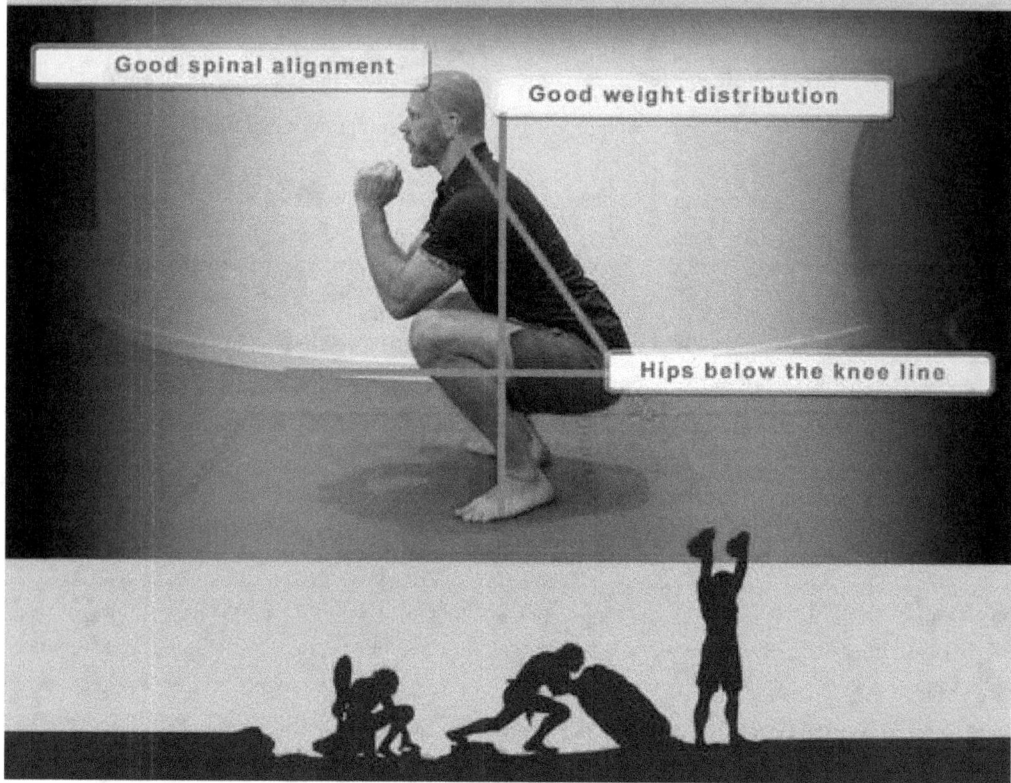


The width of the stance or angle of the feet will differ across people and yours will also change over time, it's up to you to find the right stance to start with, adjust and keep the requirements of the squat in mind as you do.

As you progress you'll be performing different depths of the squat, quarter, half, and full range. A half squat is where the hips can be seen as horizontally in line with the knees when looking side-on. There is this thing you might have heard "don't move the knees past the toes" which has become extremely popular for trainers to blurt out and sound knowledgable, forget about it, the only time you need to worry about this is if you're only moving your knees forward during the squat, i.e. knees moving forward but not counterbalancing by moving the hips back. Without a doubt, if you're maintaining good form and are getting some good depth, your knees will be moving past your toes. Back to the squat depth, you know what half a squat is, a quarter is between half and standing, and full is your maximum squat depth which should eventually be ass to grass.

# PERFECTING THE SQUAT

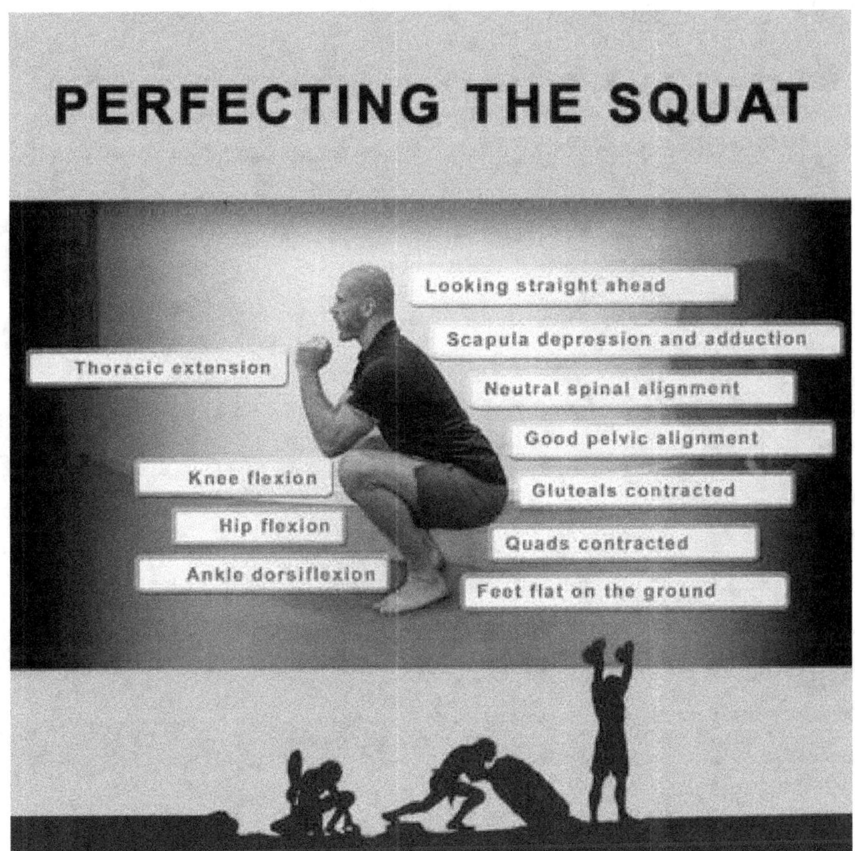



A deep squat is good for your knees. A deep squat is good for your life. Don't let anyone tell you otherwise. The only time a deep squat is bad is when it's performed incorrectly, not progressed to properly, overtraining, bad programming, you're injured or going too heavy.

# SQUAT ALIGNMENT
## PERFECTING THE SQUAT

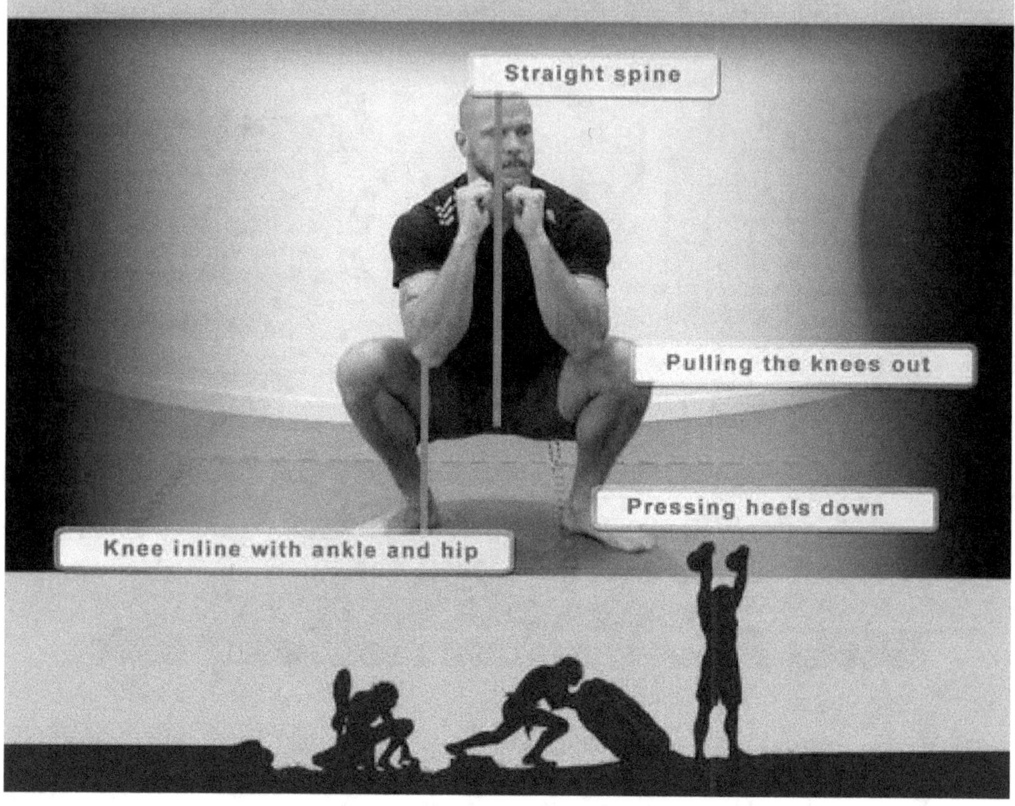


There are several things I like to say to make it clear what the objective of a squat is and usually see an immediate change in technique.

a) → Hips low and shoulders high.

b) → Hips always moving down with the shoulders following and stopping if the hips are no longer moving down.

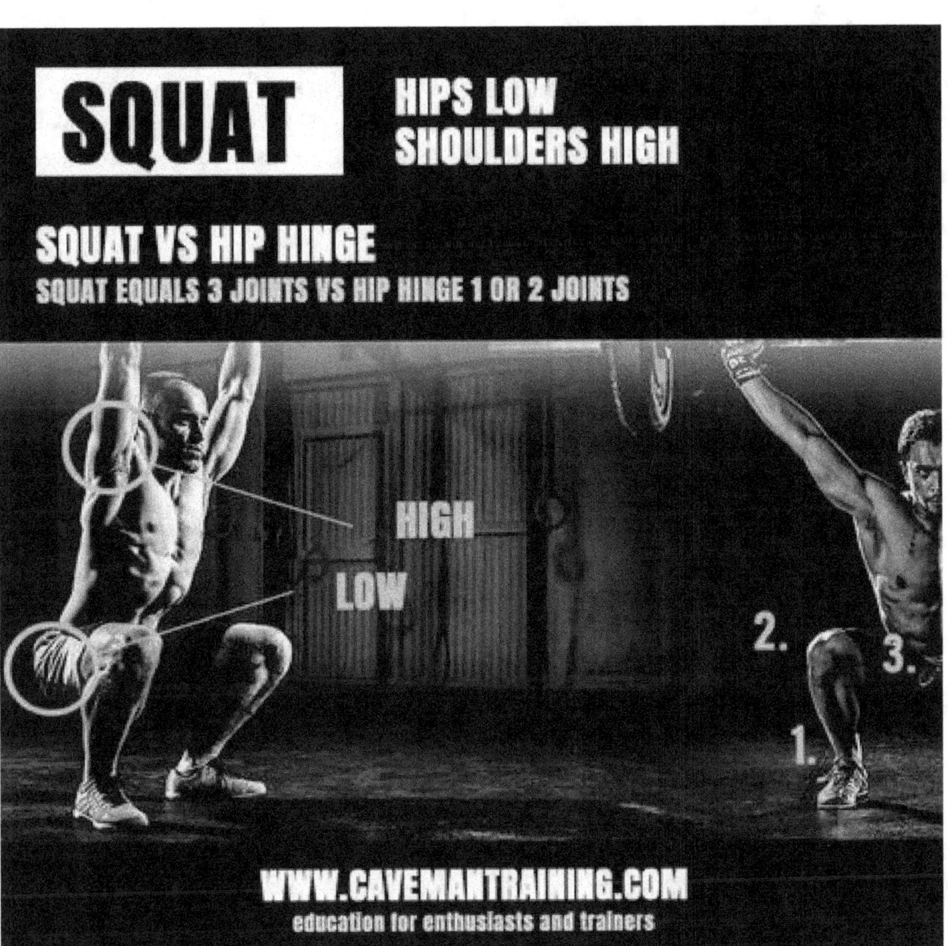
SQUAT
HIPS LOW
SHOULDERS HIGH
SQUAT VS HIP HINGE
SQUAT EQUALS 3 JOINTS VS HIP HINGE 1 OR 2 JOINTS
HIGH
LOW
2.
3.
1.
WWW.CAVEMANTRAINING.COM
education for enthusiasts and trainers

# Goblet Squat

The goblet squat is a great variation of the squat to teach the athlete how to stay upright. With the weight at the front the athlete quickly notices when he/she leans too far forward because more effort is required to hold the kettlebell up and close, and if the athlete really comes too far then the weight would pull them forward to where they fall out of the squat.

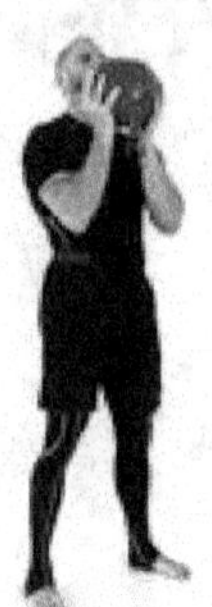
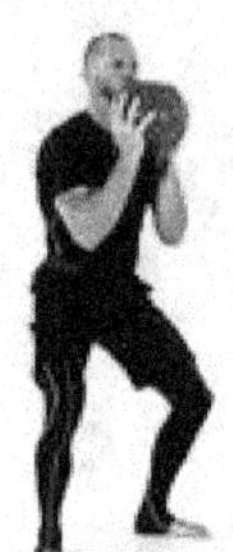
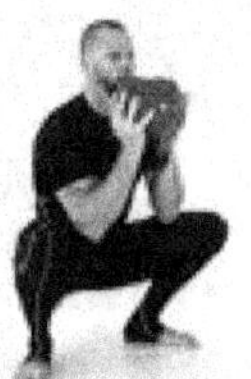
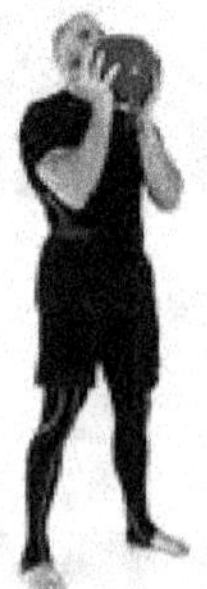
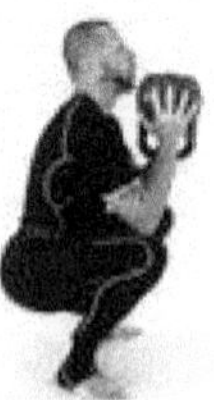

# Dead Swing Clean And Squat

*Combo*

This exercise can quite easily be turned into a clean once and multiple squats which makes it a racked squat with double kettlebells. The dead swing in this combo is great to program when you go heavy with the weights, it allows you to really focus on a slow squat which gives you more time under tension.

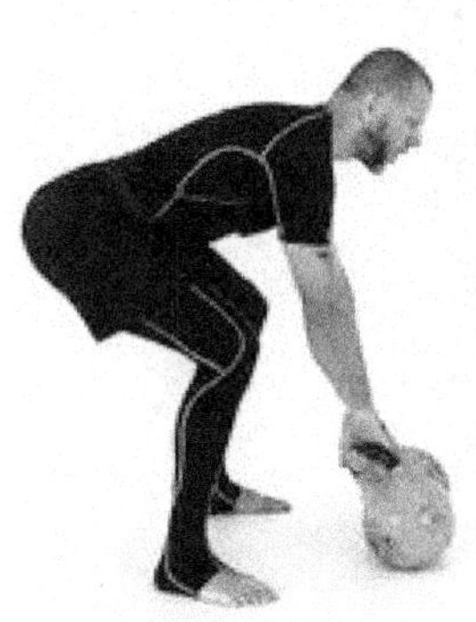 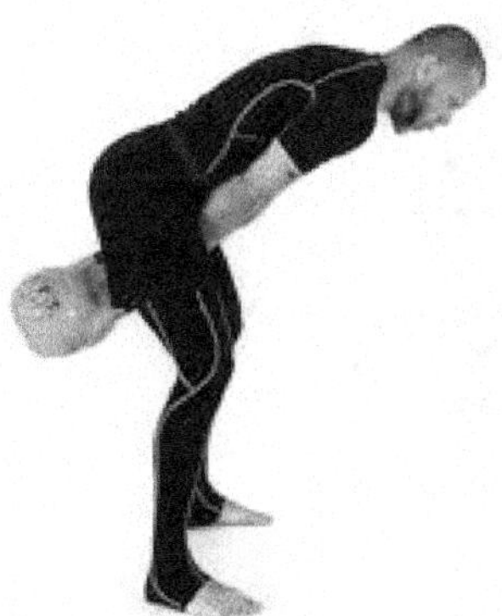

Hike the kettlebells back.

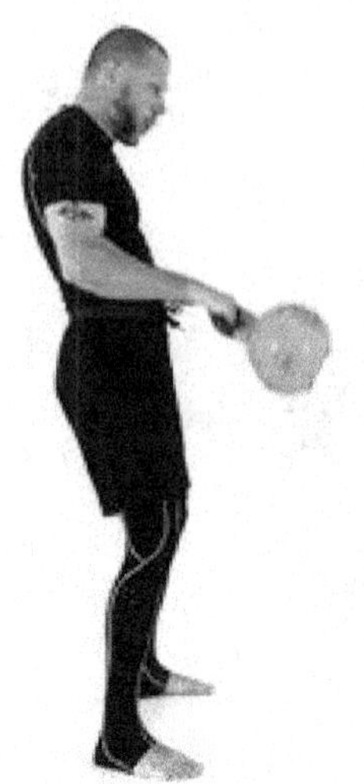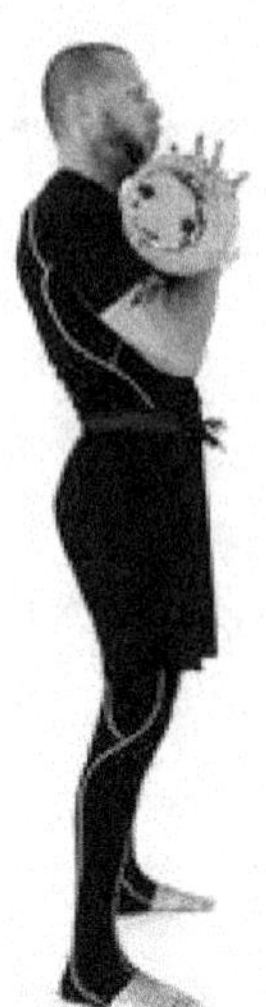

Clean the kettlebells and obtain a good racking position. Use a safety racking, flat hand, or interlocking grip to protect the fingers. The interlocking grip will make the rack easier. Easier is not always what you want from an exercise, but if you want to just focus on the squat itself, then you do.

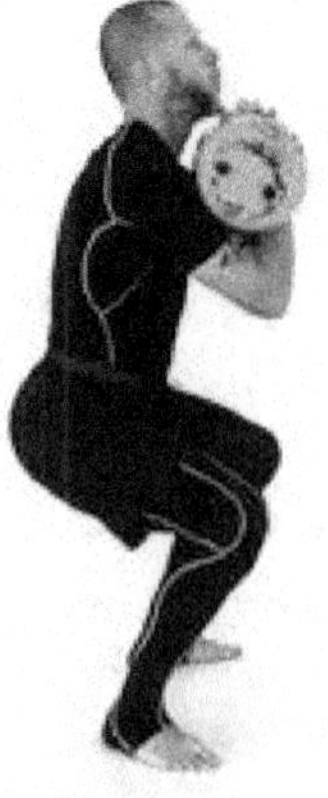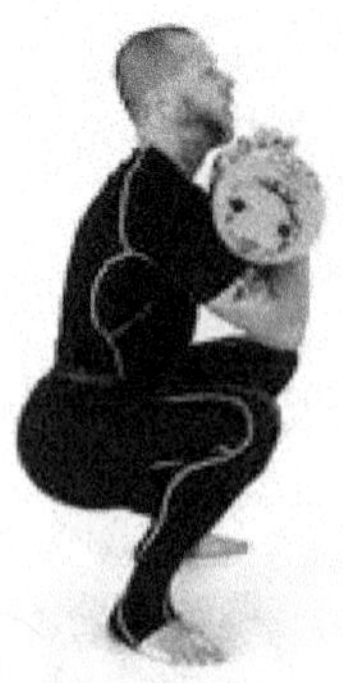

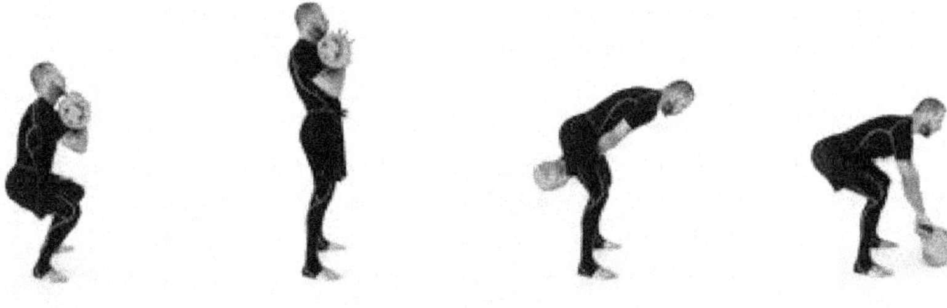

Come into full extension and return the weight to dead.

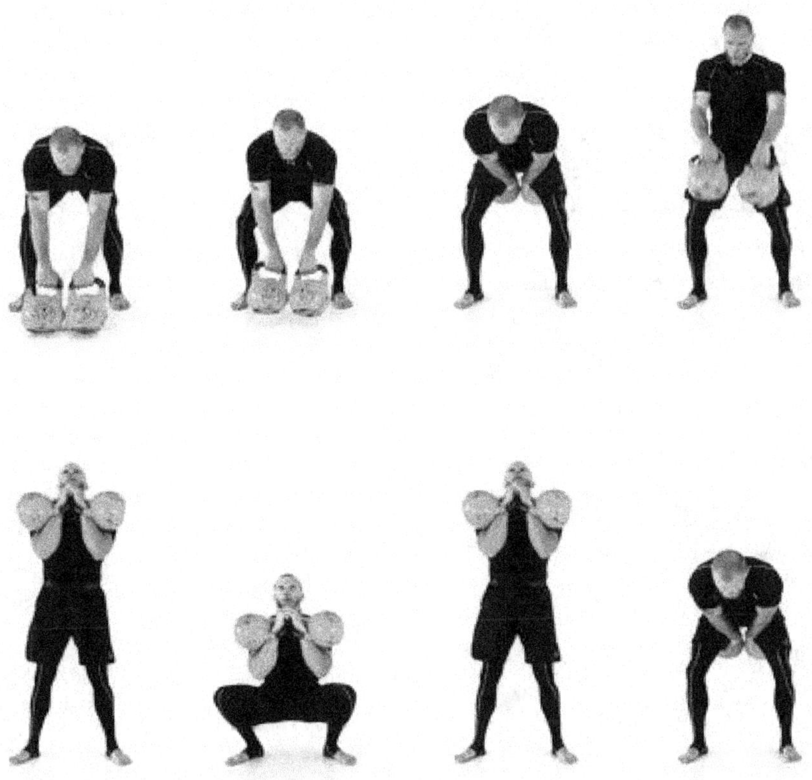

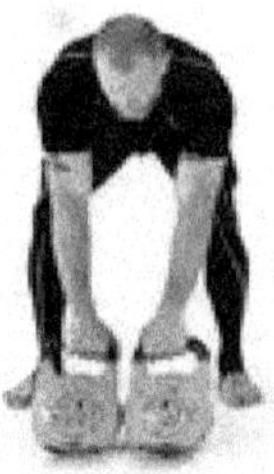

The squat itself deserves its own detailed step-by-step description and is covered in detail at the start of the squat section of this book.

**In simple terms:** The squat is flexion (one called dorsiflexion) in three joints, namely the hips, knees, and ankles, always. The second factor is the amount of flexion that dictates the depth, quarter, half, three-quarter, or full squat.

Out of the three joints, the knees are the ones providing the most flexion, and truly dictate the depth of the squat. The other two joints take care of even weight distribution.

## Squat cues

- Shoulders high and hips low
- Shoulders stop moving down when the hips do
- Push the hips toward the ground
- Look ahead
- Push the chest out
- Keep the pelvis aligned with the spine
- Adjust feet to where you're comfortable

To perform:

- Stand in a slightly wider than normal stance
- Toes slightly pointing outward

- Break at all three joints

- The knees move forward

- The hips move back and down

- The shoulders remain high

- The core is engaged

- Proper pelvic alignment should be maintained throughout the movement

- Keep looking ahead

- Maintain even weight distribution

- Maintain a neutral spine

- The feet should remain flat on the ground throughout the movement

- Move as low as is required

- Pull the knees out to keep alignment between the three squat joints

- Do not lose tension at the bottom of the squat

- Press the feet into the ground to come back up

- Contract the quadriceps for knee extension

- Contract the gluteus maximus for hip extension

- Push the heels into the ground to activate the back of the legs

- Come into full extension

## Cossack Squat

The Cossack, Curtsy lunge, and reverse lunge are literally my all-time favorite leg exercises with each providing their own awesome benefits. The Cossack squat also looks cool and you know that when you do it right, nice and deep, that everyone in the gym is jealous of you and want to come and talk to you about it.

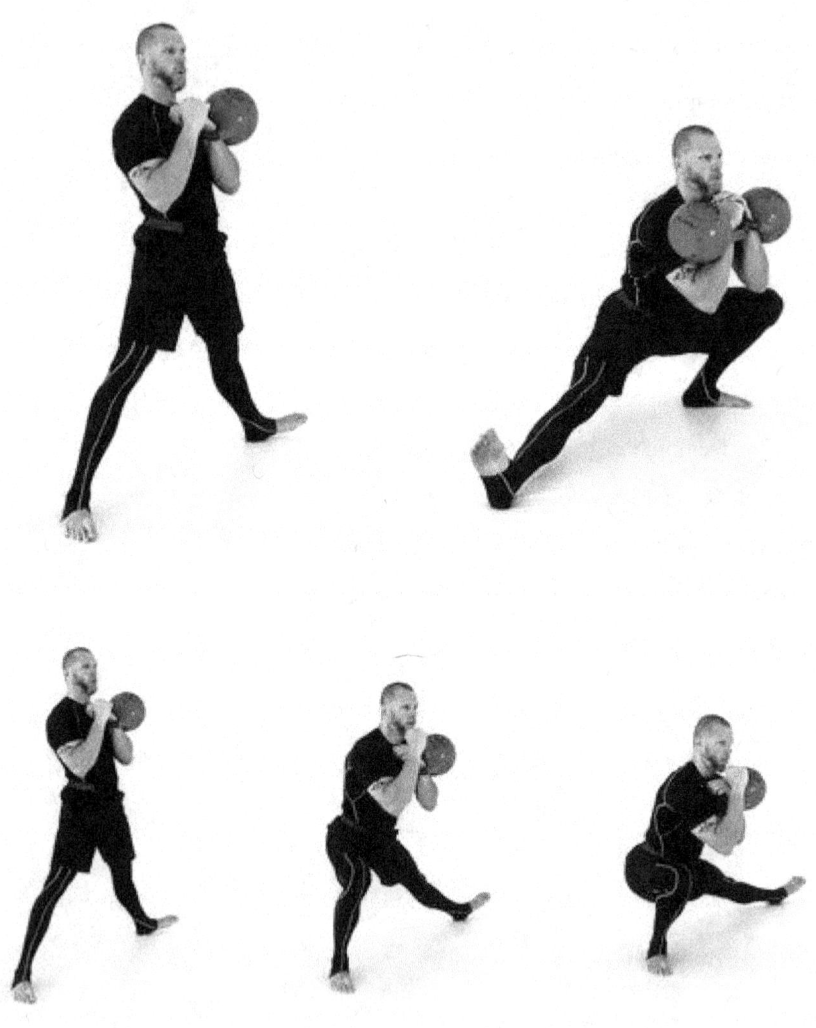

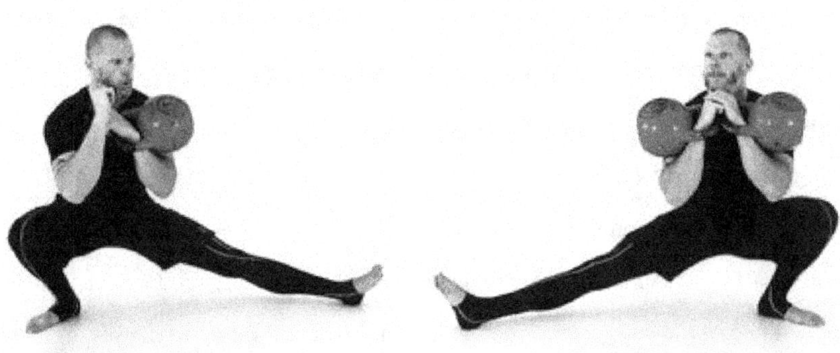

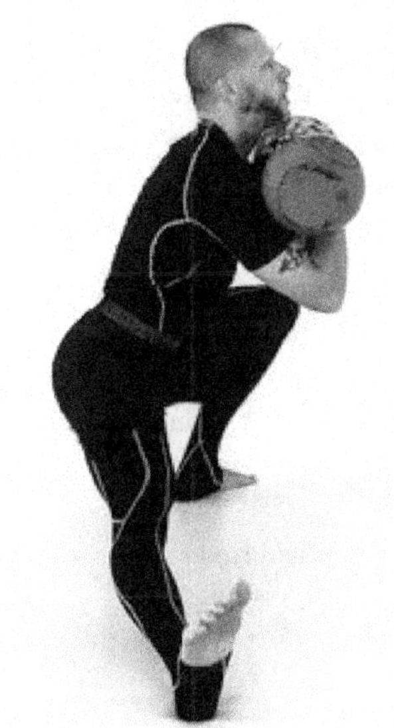

This exercise provides strength to one leg while stretching the other, and of course, the same benefits as with the regular squat apply.

The one thing that is really important with this exercise is foot placement, adjusting, and making sure you get the right angle with the foot to be able to keep moving back and down with the hips. If you get it wrong you might not be able to go deep and/or get knee problems.

**To perform:**

- Decide which leg will be the squatting leg
- Position the foot squatting leg close to the same angle as you would for a normal squat
- Don't bend the knees yet
- With the supporting leg step laterally out to the side as far as is comfortably possible
- How far you need to step out will be different for each person
- Make adjustment as you perform some reps
- Looking front on you should be making the shape of an upside-down 'Y'
- Start bending the knee on the squatting leg
- Lift the toes on the supporting side up to the sky till positioned on the heel
- Keep the knee of the supporting side locked out and pointing up to the sky
- Brace the abs
- Push the chest out and pull the shoulder blades down
- Look ahead
- Make sure to keep the joints aligned on the squatting side as you would with a normal squat
- Slowly come down while finding your balance
- Adjust the foot on the squatting side if need be
- To adjust lift the heel and then follow with the ball of the foot
- Use slow release of contraction in the quads and gluteals to come down
- Don't create fake a range by moving the shoulders further down through thoracic flexion
- Don't lose the tension once at the bottom range
- Come back up by raising the shoulders first
- Follow through with the rest of the body

You can repeat the same side or alternate. The width of the stance is the same for the other side, whether you can transition smoothly into the next squat or not will depend on how you're able to angle that foot during the transition.

**Benefits:**

1. Strength

2. Progression to pistol squats

3. Stability

4. Flexibility

5. Isolation


One of the issues I commonly see is the foot on the squatting leg is turned out too much which means that the hips are stopped from going further down because instead, they're going in the direction of the supporting leg which is not moving. To come further down with the hips they need to be able to move back and down just like with a normal squat, hence, the foot needs to be angled in such a way it will allow natural and safe movement in that direction.


The Cossack squat is a great progression to the pistol squat. The pistol squat was an exercise I looked at ages ago and knew that it was great for strength and stability, but what about functional? Not that everything has to be functional, on the contrary, but it's always fun to know how it could be. In the case of the pistol squat, I quickly found out how it helped me enjoy a holiday more than I otherwise would have while I had my leg in a cast after a deep cut in my ankle. We were camping around Xmas time on the Sunshine Coast in Queensland when this happened and I did not want it to ruin the families together time. Anyways, being able to easily get up with one leg due to training pistol squats paid off and is functional.

# Fireman's Squat

AKA back squat

This is the kettlebell version of the barbell back squat. To get the kettlebells in the racking position you will need to press them overhead first and then lower them into position. The benefit of this squat variation is that the weight is higher, directly positioned above the center of gravity, and does not require much shoulder or arm work, that is if the kettlebells are positioned correctly with the round part of the bell resting on the trapezius.

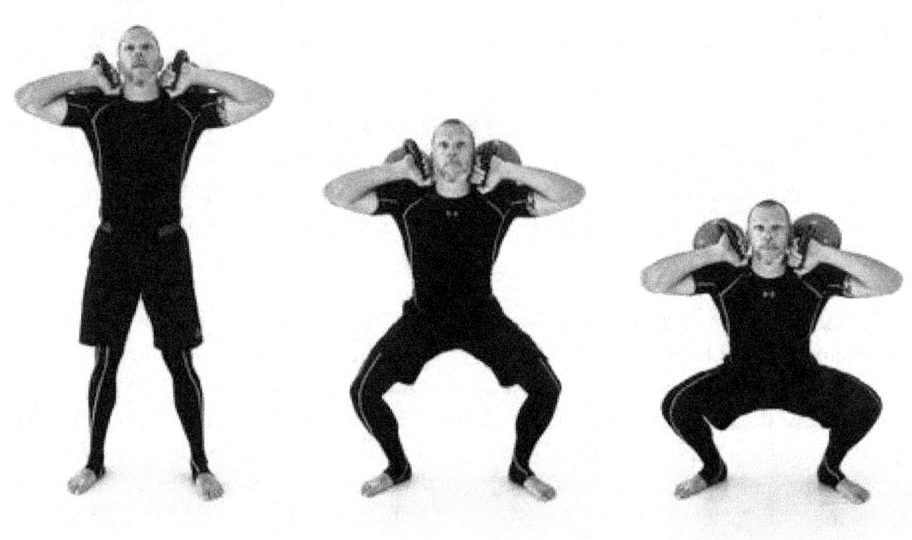

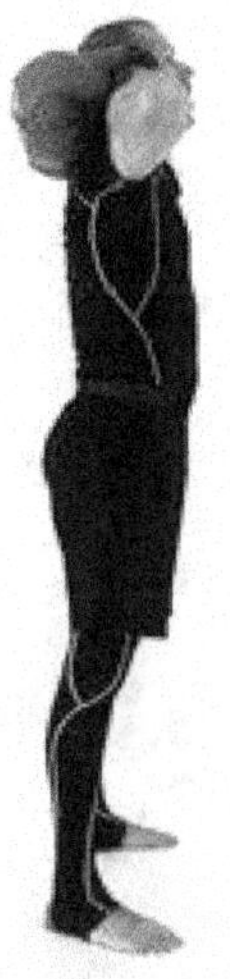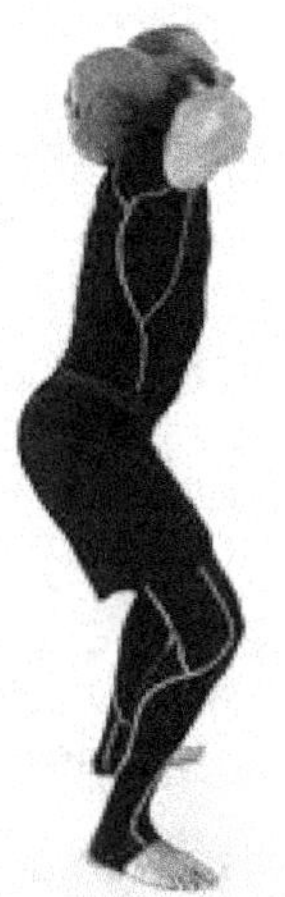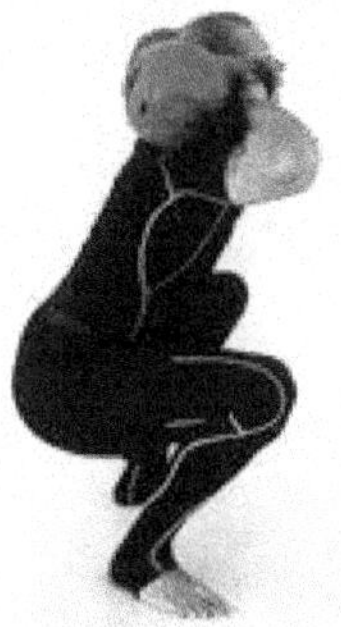

# Racked Squat

AKA: Front squat

The racked squat simply requires a clean and a good racking position. You can interlace the fingers (interlocked grip) for stability and making the rack easier, which allows you to focus more on the squat itself. You want to keep the elbows under the weight as you squat. The great thing about a racked squat is that it requires you to stay upright, if you come forward to far then the weight will be pulling you forward and out of balance.

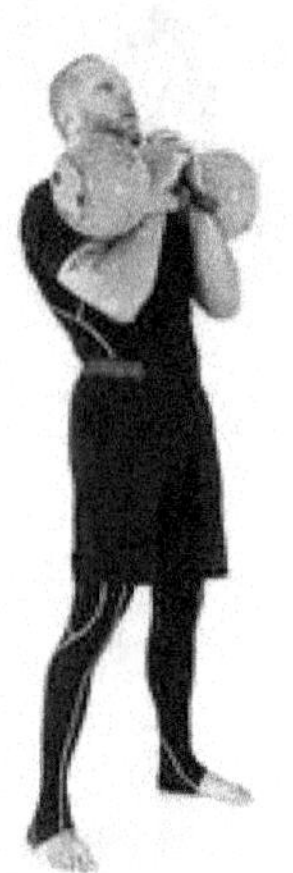 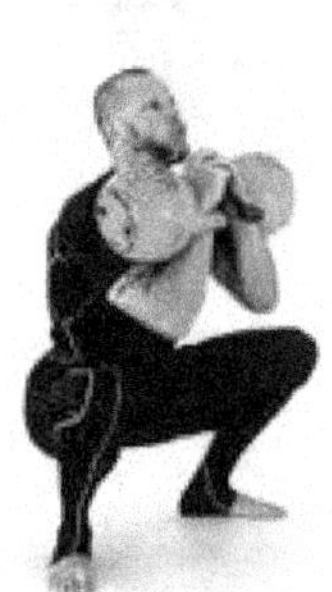 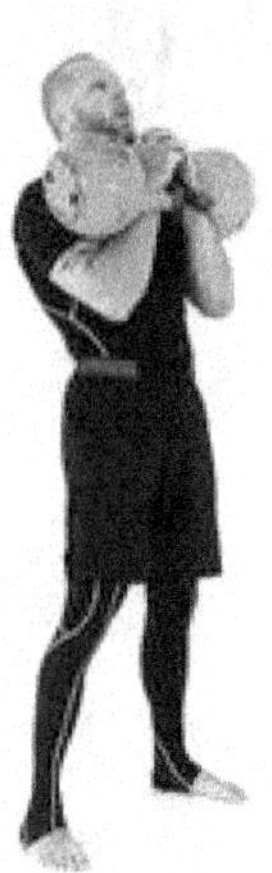

You can use one or two kettlebells for the racked squat. Using one kettlebell challenges the stabilizers more. You can keep them racked and for example for strength doing 6 to 8 slow deep reps in a minute and then rest 30 to 60 seconds. You can also make it more dynamic and keep the dead swing clean in, i.e. clean and squat upon each rep. The sequence below demonstrates the dead swing squat and back to dead.

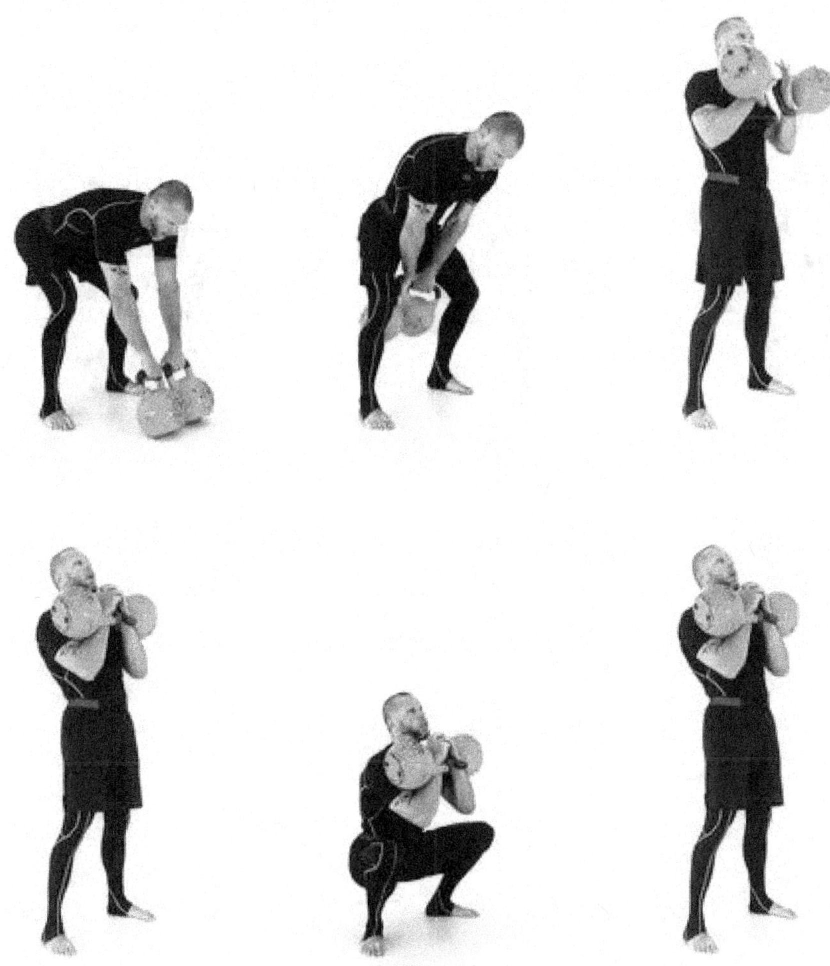

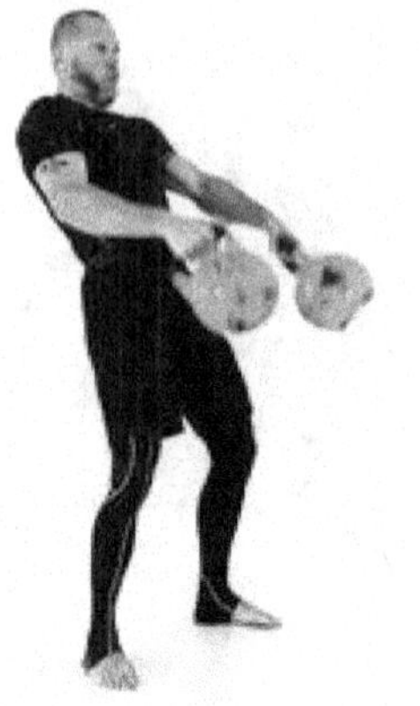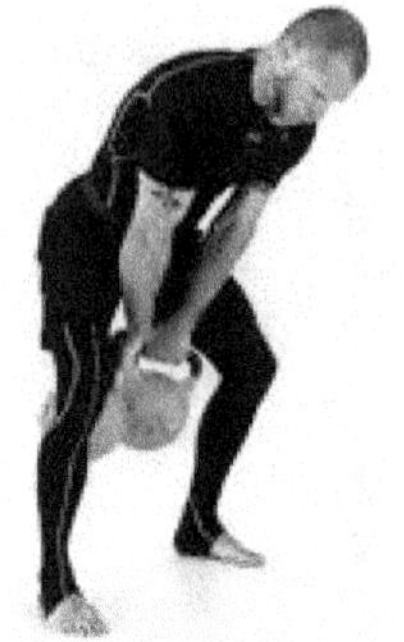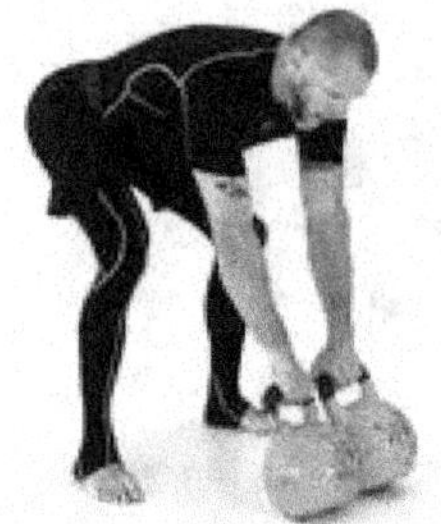

## Overhead Squat

AKA: OH squat

The overhead squat with kettlebells is a lot harder than the barbell overhead squat due to the kettlebell being unilateral, you can't pull the bar apart for stability, and the weight needs to be placed right above your shoulder. For a good overhead squat, you need good shoulder mobility and strength. You also need strength in the back to keep it upright, or rather more than upright and create thoracic hyperextension. If you don't then the shoulder needs to do more work or won't be able to keep the weight up overhead.

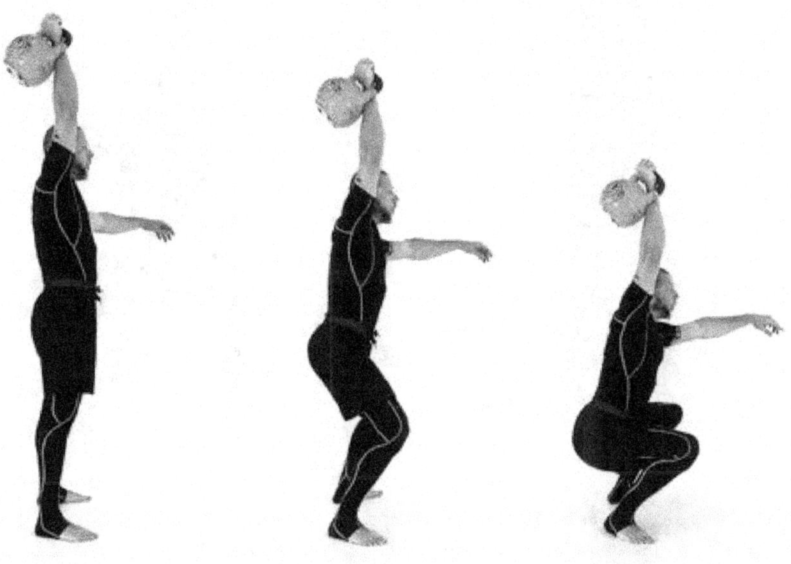

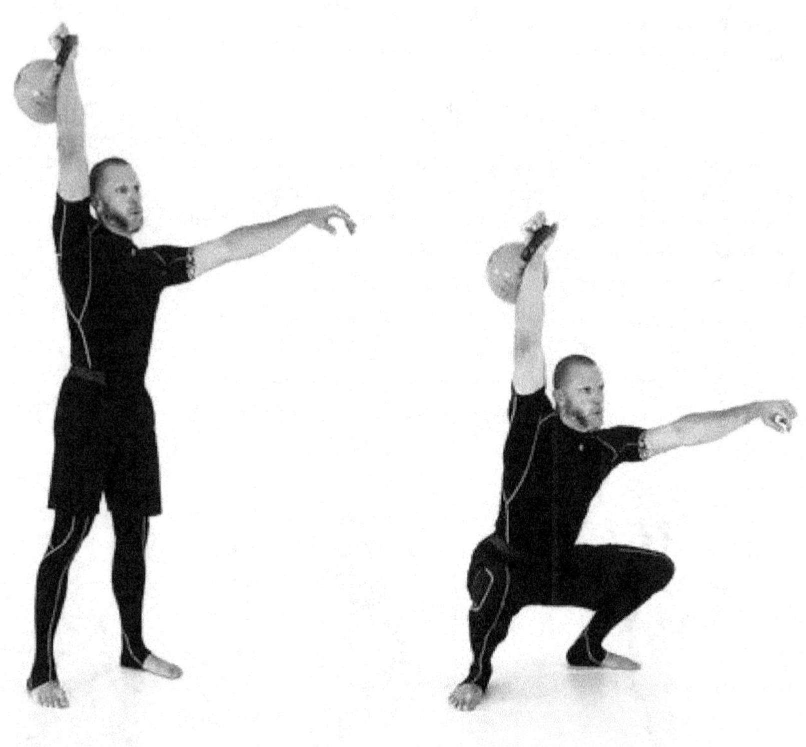

When doing single overhead squats you will notice that a lot of work needs to be done on the non-lifting side to stabilize the torso (spine). Before you descent into the overhead squat you want to create tension through the body and especially those areas that you'll feel pull in the deepest part of the squat. Do not force a deep overhead squat, it can cause injury injury in the shoulders, and/or internally, like the quadratus lumborum which will have to work hard to prevent lateral flexion of the spine.

## Racked Overhead Squat

The racked overhead squat is a progression to the double kettlebell overhead squat, but also just great to add additional weight to the single arm overhead squat. The great things is that the racked kettlebell will take away that pull on the quadratus lumborum (QL) in the non-overhead side. Hence, a great variation to use if you've been trying the single overhead squat and found that it became uncomfortable in the QL.

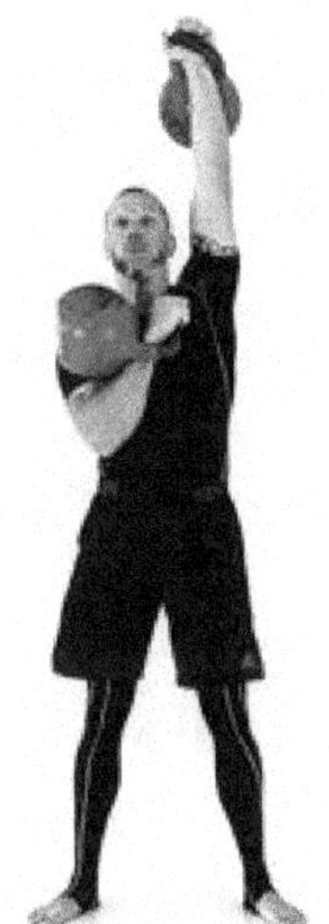
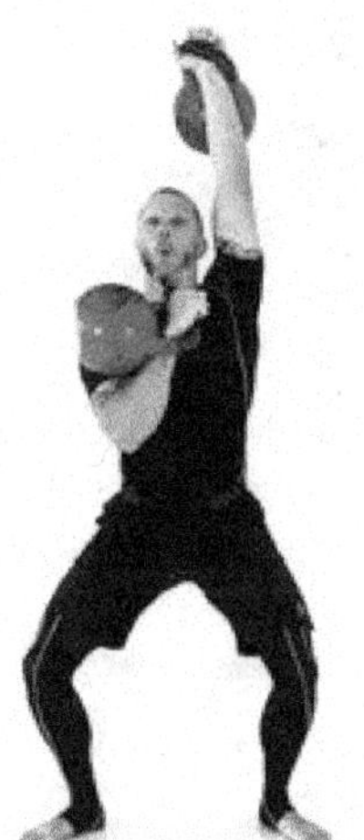
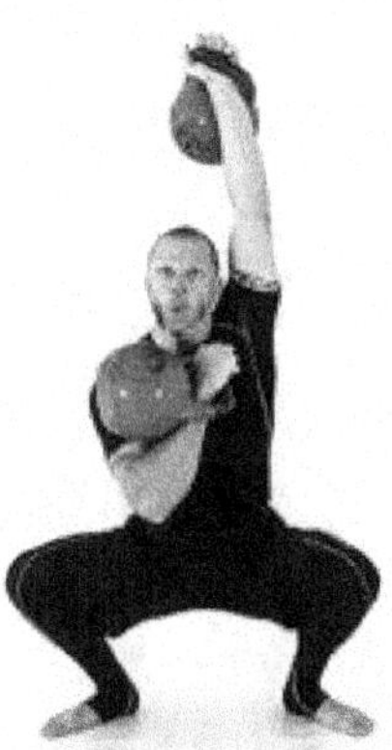

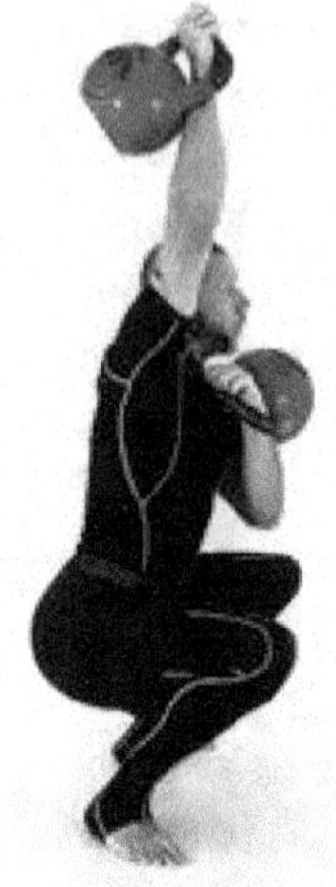

## Frontal Hold Squat

The frontal hold squat is part isometric and part dynamic, the hold is isometric and the squat is dynamic. You can make it a totally isometric exercise by staying in the bottom position, but not resting in the position, stopping just before hitting max relaxed depth. This exercise works the deltoids and upper back plus everything from a normal squat.

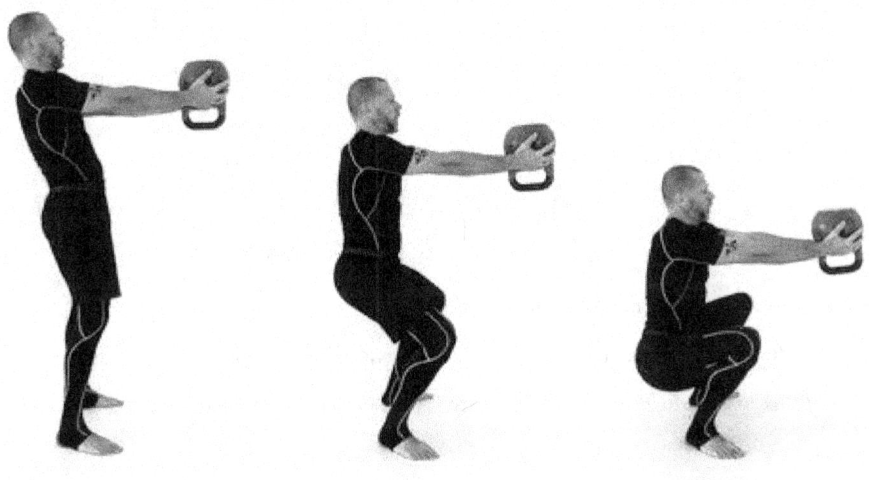

# Hindu Squat

This exercise is by no means a beginner exercise, it's an advanced exercise everyone should work up to. It's not only great for strength in the quads but also extremely good for the balls of the feet, but there is so much more you get from it, for example, calf strength, your stabilization is challenged, and you can expect increased ankle flexibility.

**To perform:**

- Stand in a neutral stance

- Come on to the balls of your feet by contracting the calves and pulling the heels off the ground

- Find your balance

- Torso remains straight and vertically aligned throughout the whole movement

- Hips and shoulders remain above the ankles when viewed side on

- Press the balls of the feet into the ground

- Contract your quads to control the knee flexion that follows

- Break at the knees and let them come forward in a controlled manner

- Create more dorsiflexion in the ankles as you come down

- Slowly lower to the bottom position

- Come back up by pulling the knees back in through ankle plantar flexion, knee and hip extension

- The heels never touch the ground

The Hindu squat requires a lot of quad and calf strength before you attempt the exercise, starting this exercise without that strength is going to cause injury without a doubt. If you experience pain around the knee area, re-asses your strength.

Before you attempt the Hindu squat with kettlebells you should master the exercise with just bodyweight, after that you can add one racked kettlebell, two racked kettlebells, one kettlebell overhead, one kettlebell overhead and one racked, and ultimately two kettlebells overhead. The Hindu squat is more difficult than a normal squat but the overhead Hindu squat is easier than the overhead squat as the spine can remain completely straight during a Hindu squat whereas with a normal squat the shoulders are pulled forward (depending on overall flexibility).

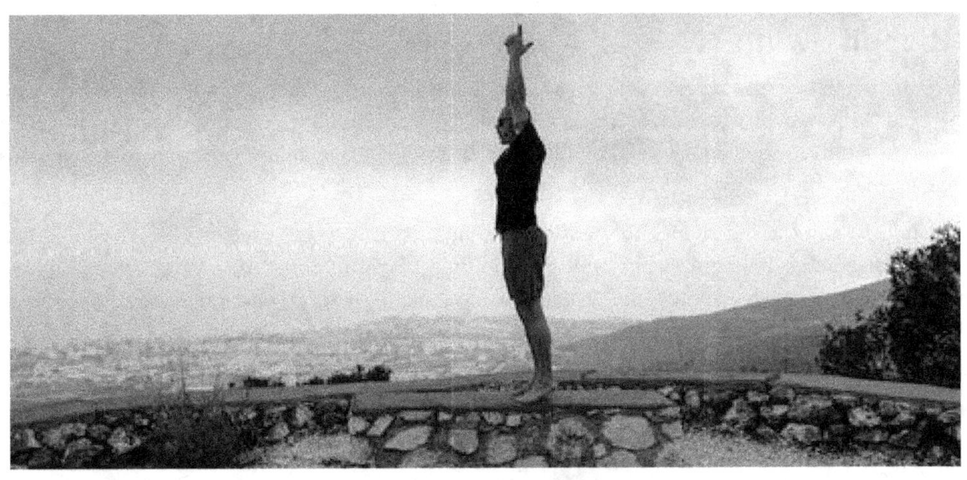

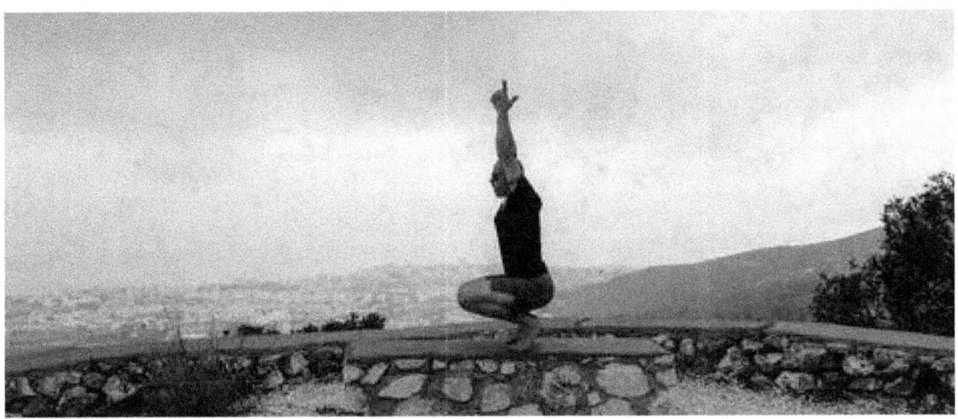

**Bonus videos:**
Bodyweight Hindu Squat go.cavemantraining.com/kbe-vid-129
Double Kettlebell Overhead Hindu Squat go.cavemantraining.com/kbe-vid-130

# Kettlebell Swing

Kettlebell swings are an exercise where a weight swings back and forth or from side to side while being held with one or two hands. The swing can be performed with many different movement patterns, hip hinge, squat, and pendulum. From there you have many other attributes that can change up the swing.

In general, if you're doing swings for cardio or strength then you will be doing them fast and want as much resistance from them, hence, you'll be pulling. If you're doing the swing for endurance or sport, then you want to employ the pendulum movement (natural+push) and remove as much resistance as possible while going with the flow.

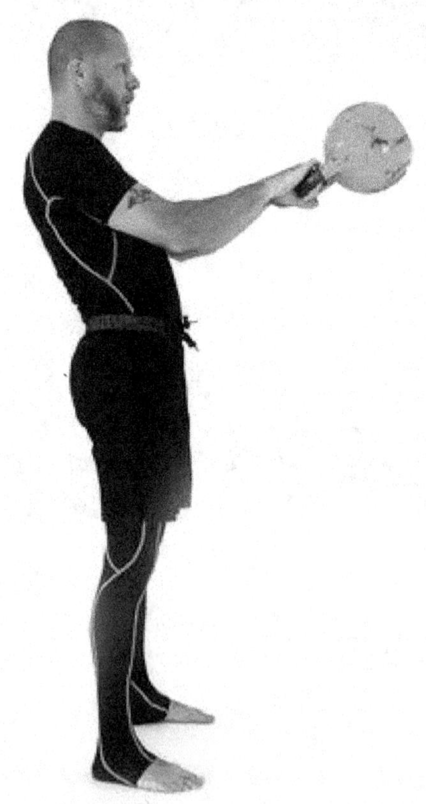

## Starting The Swing

There are three common ways to start the swing. The first is dead from the ground. The second is from hang and bump, this is performed by standing in a neutral position with the bell hanging and positioned above the thigh, moving the thigh slightly back and bumping the weight out into the first swing. The third is from racking position straight into swinging.

## Ending The Swing

How you end your swing is just as important as how you start it. There are two common ways to end the swing, the first is bringing it back dead to the ground in reverse order of how you started it with a dead swing. The second is by cleaning the bell up and then racking or returning straight to the ground.

## American Swing

The American swing can be performed a hip hinge or squat style, the main difference is that the arms should end up overhead and locked out with the base of the kettlebell pointing up.

Note the following differences compared to the other swing variations:

1.  More power needs to be generated to propel the kettlebell higher

2.  The direction of the kettlebell should be up rather than forward and up

3.  Shoulders will be involved to get the kettlebell overhead and locked-out

4.  The most efficient way to get the kettlebell up and down is the shortest path

5.  The shortest path is keeping the bell closer to the body and pressing out

6.  Arms can bend on the up and down phase

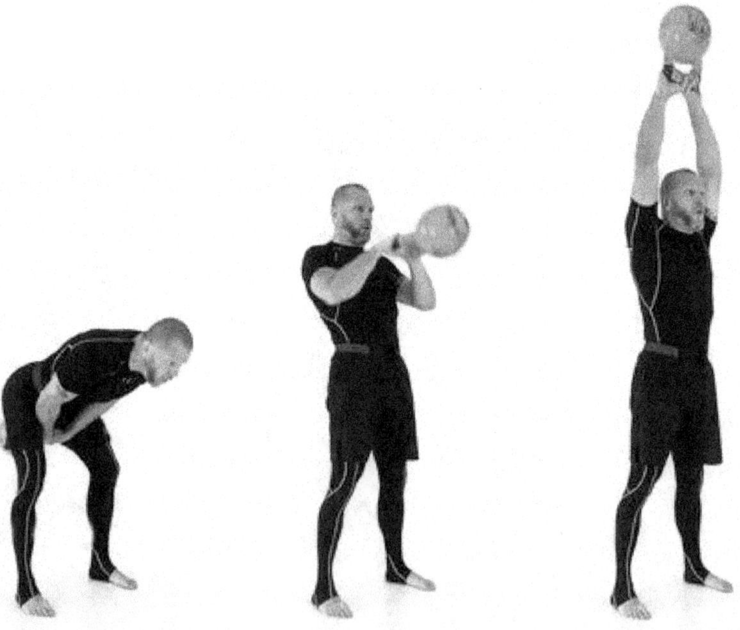

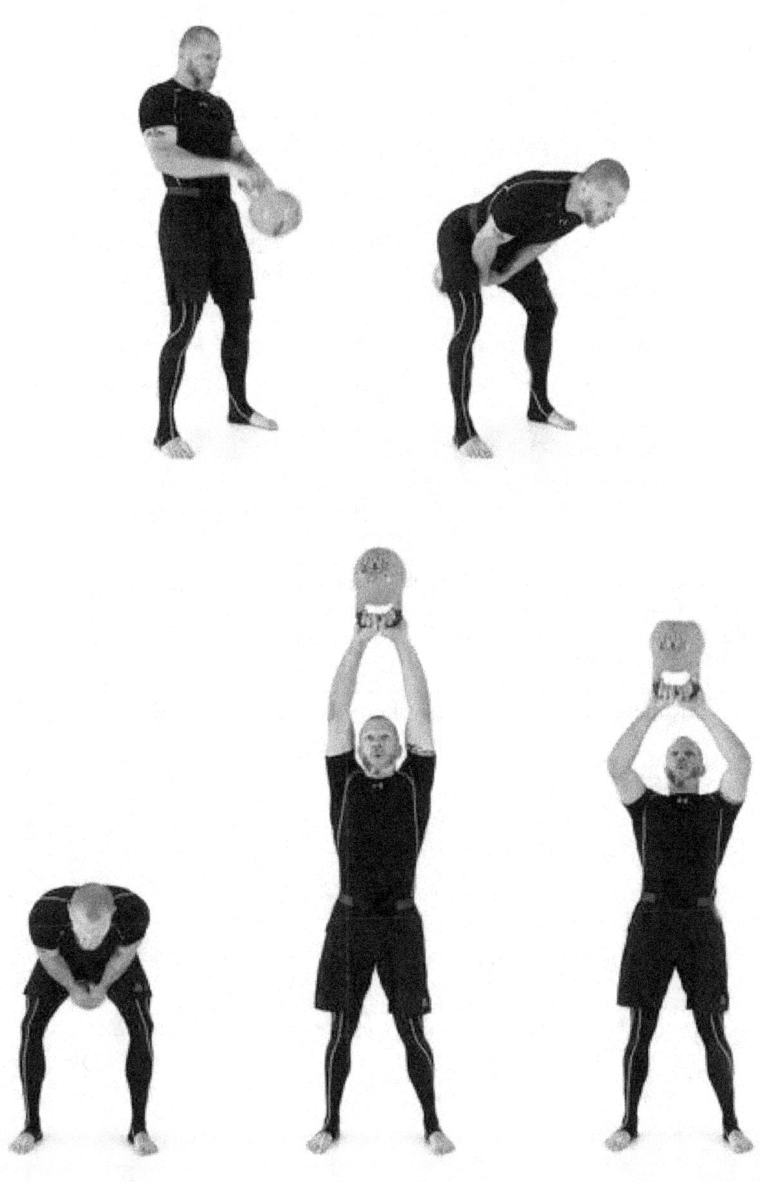

It should be noted that arms straight throughout the movement are going to give you the most results from this resistance training exercise. Keeping the arms straight will also require more shoulder involvement, which is a good thing if that's what you want to train. On the other side there is competition, in which it's all about meeting movement standards and how you get there in between or whether you take shortcuts usually does not matter.

To perform:

- Perform a swing

- Follow through with a shoulder raise

- Lock the arms out overhead

- Let the bell drop back with slightly bent arms to keep the drop closer

- Guide into the backswing and repeat

You can also replace the raise with a press out and treat this as a double arm snatch.

Dot points:

- The American swing is a swing that does involve a shoulder raise

- This version of the swing is created by CrossFit

- Before you do this exercise you need to check if you can safely/easily bring your arms above your head with a close grip

- The American swing is great if you want to work your shoulders and legs at the same time

- The swing can be performed with a squat, hip hinge, or pendulum

*I personally prefer double bell snatches.*

*go.cavemantraining.com/double-kb-snatch*

## Gorilla Swings

Gorilla swings are great to keep tension on the legs throughout the movement, as you're swinging back your whole posterior stretches, and as you move into the squat and swing the weight away from you, you will need to keep full tension in the legs and back to create a solid base to control that weight. I prefer to do these to work on flexibility in the hamstrings, back-strength, and stability.

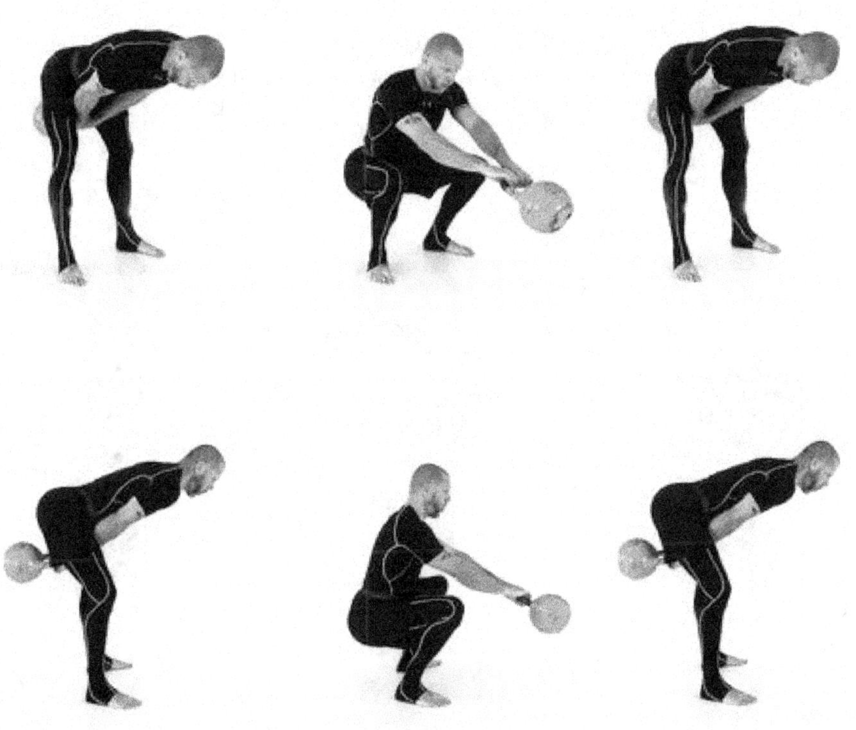

Really try and get those legs as straight as possible on the backswing for that stretch, but make sure you progress appropriately. You require good coordination as you swing forward while you move into the squat.

# Hip Hinge Swing

## Single Kettlebell Double Arm

AKA: Russian swing, conventional swing.

**Conventional**: Based on or in accordance with what is generally done or believed.

It should be noted that although this is referred to as the conventional swing, this is only due to this movement is what popularized the kettlebell swing and is the most common variation of the swing seen outside of sport. If you'd wanted to look at this from the perspective of what variation of the swing came first, then it would be the pendulum swing from kettlebell sport, which was used in Russia way before the kettlebell swing became popular outside of Russia.

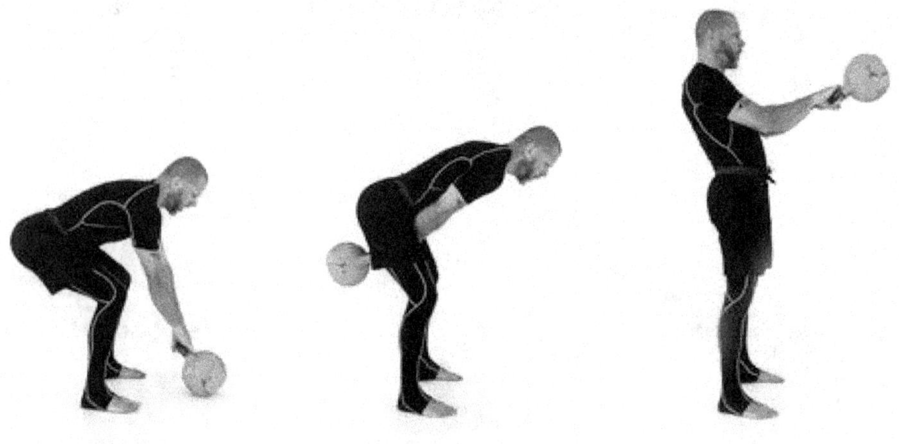

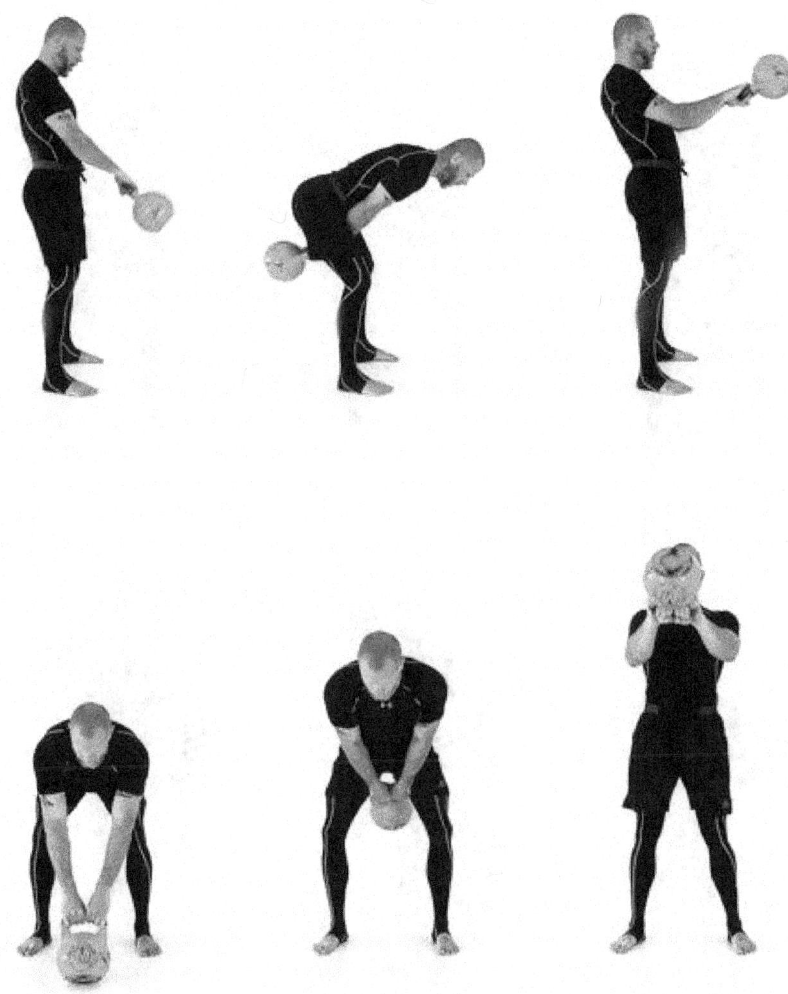

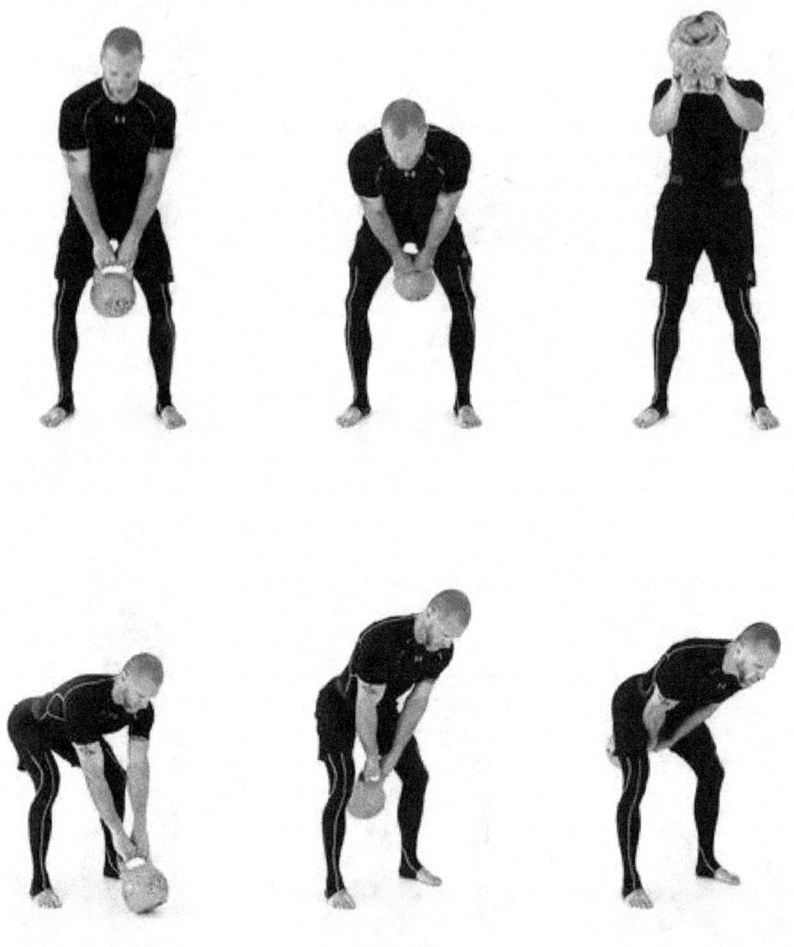

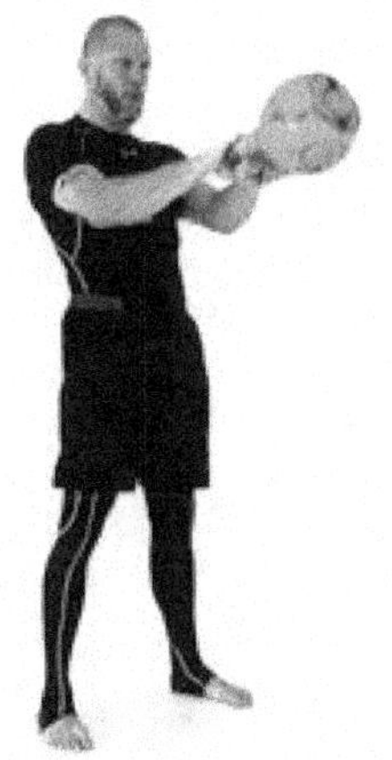 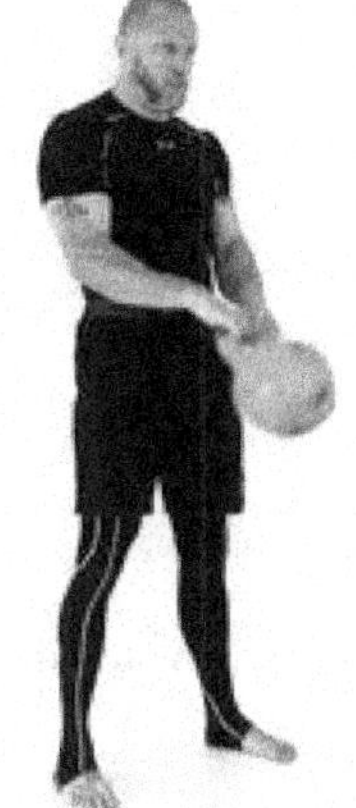 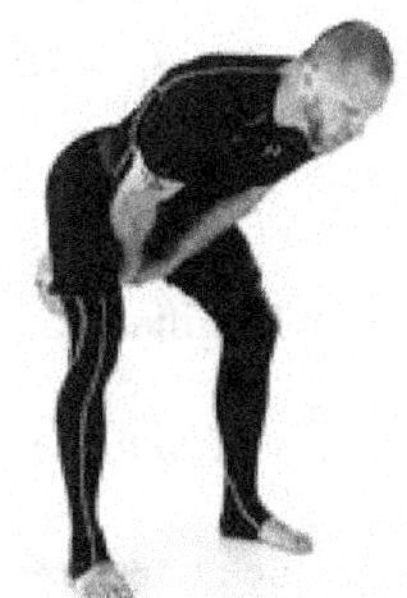

To perform the double-arm swing with one kettlebell:

1. **START OF THE SWING** Stand in a neutral position

2. Feet slightly wider than shoulder-width

3. Kettlebell placed in-front of you

4. Maintain a neutral spine and a braced core

5. Maintain flat feet on the ground

6. Maintain straight arms
   *(this can change once you've mastered the swing)*

7. Maintain relaxed shoulders

8. Think of the arms as a rod and shoulders as a pivot

9. Hip hinge and reach for the kettlebell
   (do not overreach)

10. Grab the kettlebell by the handle with both hands and a loose grip

11. Create slight tension between yourself and the kettlebell

12. Pull the kettlebell off the ground and hike it back through the legs

13. Slightly bring the shoulders up during the pull from the ground and into the backswing

14. The height at which the kettlebell comes through should be around knee height

15. Elbows making a connection with the belly around the first ribs of the ribcage

16. The outside of the wrist making a connection or being around the inside thigh area

17. Direct the kettlebell to the back

18. **UPSWING** Initiate the pull-out

19. Press the heels into the ground with weight evenly distributed across the foot

20. Contract the gluteus maximus to pull the pelvis up and propel the bell forward

21. Contract the hamstring muscles to assist in pulling the pelvis up

22. Follow through with an explosive but controlled full hip extension

23. Full knee extension

24. The whole body comes into full extension

25. The power from the lower-body; and the upper-body coming upright is what propels the kettlebell

26. Do not lean back at the lumbar to pull the weight higher
    *(proper hip hyperextension is different and might be required when working with heavyweights to create counterbalance)*

27. **FLOAT**
    The top of the swing is when the kettlebell is motionless in the air for a split second

28. The kettlebell only needs to swing as high as the force generated by your lower-body will move it; which is usually about chest height

29. At the top of the swing remember:

    - Chest out

    - Shoulders back

    - Latissimus dorsi pulled down

- Core braced

- Gluteals squeezed

- Legs are straight

- Look ahead

30. **BACKSWING** Get ready to break at the hips when the kettlebell starts to fall down

31. Delay breaking of the hips as long as possible to prevent unbalancing the movement
*(the heavier the weight or the more fatigue is present the longer the delay)*

32. The kettlebell should come through the legs approximately around the knees
*(you should be able to put another kettlebell between your legs and not hit it)*

33. Perform an insert and push the weight through

34. Elbows/forearms should be making contact around the waistline

35. You should feel the tension on the hamstrings when pushing the hips back

36. Remember that **this version** of the swing is not a squat

37. **REPEAT UPSWING**

## The hip hinge

- hip flexion paired with knee flexion
- hips moving back and slightly down
- knees remain positioned above the ankles/shins vertical
- no ankle dorsiflexion
- shoulders come toward the ground
- approximately 45 to 60 degrees of flexion in the hips and knees
- followed by extension in the hips and knees
- coming into full extension

## Breathing

You can inhale on the down-phase and exhale on the up-phase. You can inhale through the nose and out through the mouth or do both through the mouth. You can forcefully breathe out through the mouth when up or down, the inhale happens automatically during the movement. Whatever breathing pattern you choose, do not hold your breath during the swing.

## Muscles worked

Hip hinge swing which means you prevent movement in your ankles, there is flexion and extension in the knees and hips. A full step-by-step description of the movement is further down.

The kettlebell swing is a full-body exercise that uses muscles for grip, posture, stabilization, to keep the spine erect, and the actual movement (prime movers). I cover the two-handed swing, the single-handed swing would involve a lot more action around the mid-section.

## Grip

- Flexor digitorum superficialis
- Flexor digitorum profundus
- Flexor digit minimi brevis
- Lumbricals

## Posture/shoulders

- Rhomboideus minor
- Rhomboideus major
- Lower trapezius
- Levator scapulae
- Latissimus dorsi

## Spine

- Iliocostalis
- Longissimus
- Spinalis

## Prime movers

- Gluteus maximus

* Bicep femoris (long head)

* Semitendinosus

* Semimembranosus

## Flexion and stabilization

* Biceps femoris

* Semitendinosus

* Semimembranosus

* Gracilis

* Sartorius

* Gastrocnemius

* Soleus

* Popliteus

## Grip

The muscles used for grip are usually not mentioned or thought off, however, your swing is only as good as your grip. In fact, most of your training is only as good as your grip, if you have a weak grip then you won't be lifting heavy. If your grip has no endurance then you won't be completing high reps unbroken.

## Posture/shoulders

I'm referring to the top part of your body at the top of the swing where your shoulders are nice and safely pulled down. Your chest it out, shoulders blades slightly down and pulled together.

## Spine

Throughout the swing, your erector spinae muscles need to work to keep your spine erect, and there is actually a lot more going on inside as well to protect the spine and brace the abs.

## Prime movers

These are the muscles that create the movement which is the hip and knee extension only when we're talking about the conventional kettlebell swing.

## Flexion and stabilization

The flexion I refer to is knee flexion and the stabilization I refer to is that of keeping the knee in place above the ankle. Keeping the knee above the ankle is important when hip hinging, if the knee comes excessively forward, then the movement starts to turn into a squat. A kettlebell squat swing is not bad, it's only bad if you need to perform a hip hinge and perform a squat, or perform the squat swing incorrectly, otherwise, the squat swing is an excellent exercise. See a side by side comparison of the hip hinge versus squat swing.

## Safety

A key safety point to consider. Don't follow the kettlebell, protect the lower back! A video about this is included in the bonus material that you can view online. At the top of the swing when the kettlebell is going back down you do not want to follow it and break at the hips the same time the kettlebell goes back down, this will put a lot of pressure on the lower back, instead, wait for the kettlebell to be at a good height to create hip flexion and keep the back safe. A good height is usually when the bell is or nears the legs.

## Single Kettlebell Single Arm

When you work with one arm instead of two there is more load to work with but there is also more pull on the torso, a rotational pull that would rotate the spine if you did not resist it. That same rotational pull does not exist when working with double-arm. Either variation has its own benefits. A great thing about the single-arm swing is that it is the foundation for the clean and snatch.

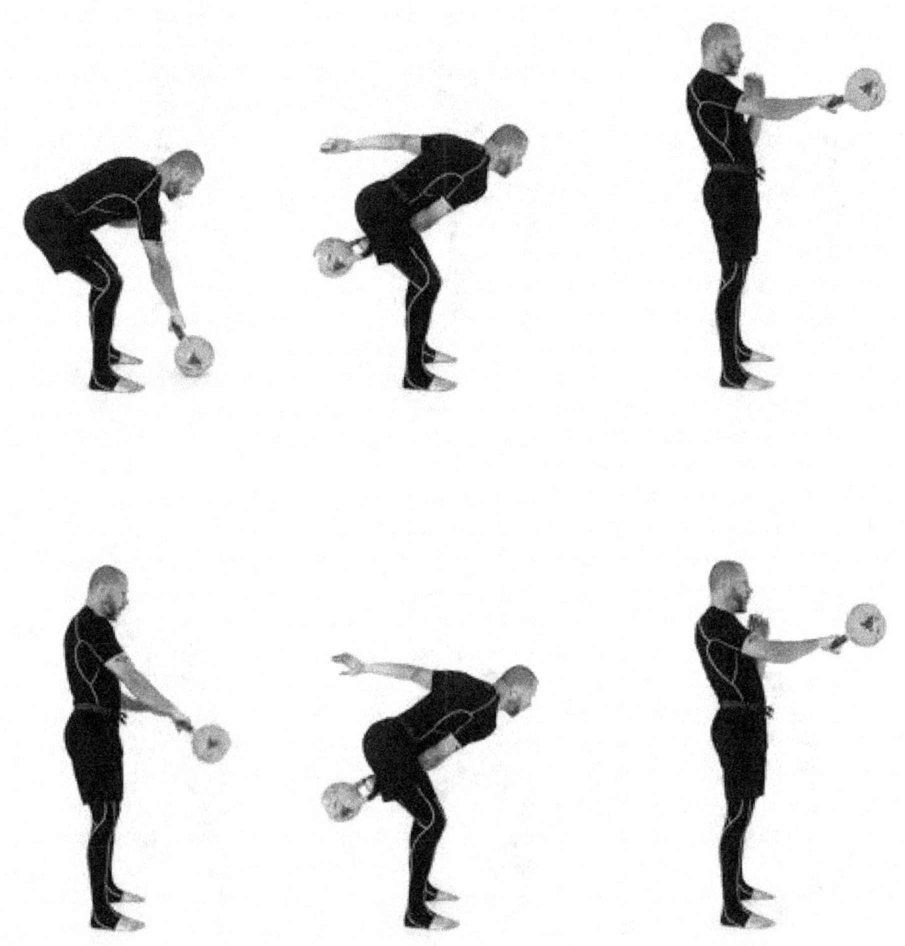

You can swing and resist the rotational pull on the spine or you can go with it and let thoracic rotation happen. If you want to go with the flow then you would let the thoracic rotation happen on the down phase/backswing, not on the upswing, at least not for this type of swing. If you were doing cleans you could create rotation to pull the kettlebell in more.

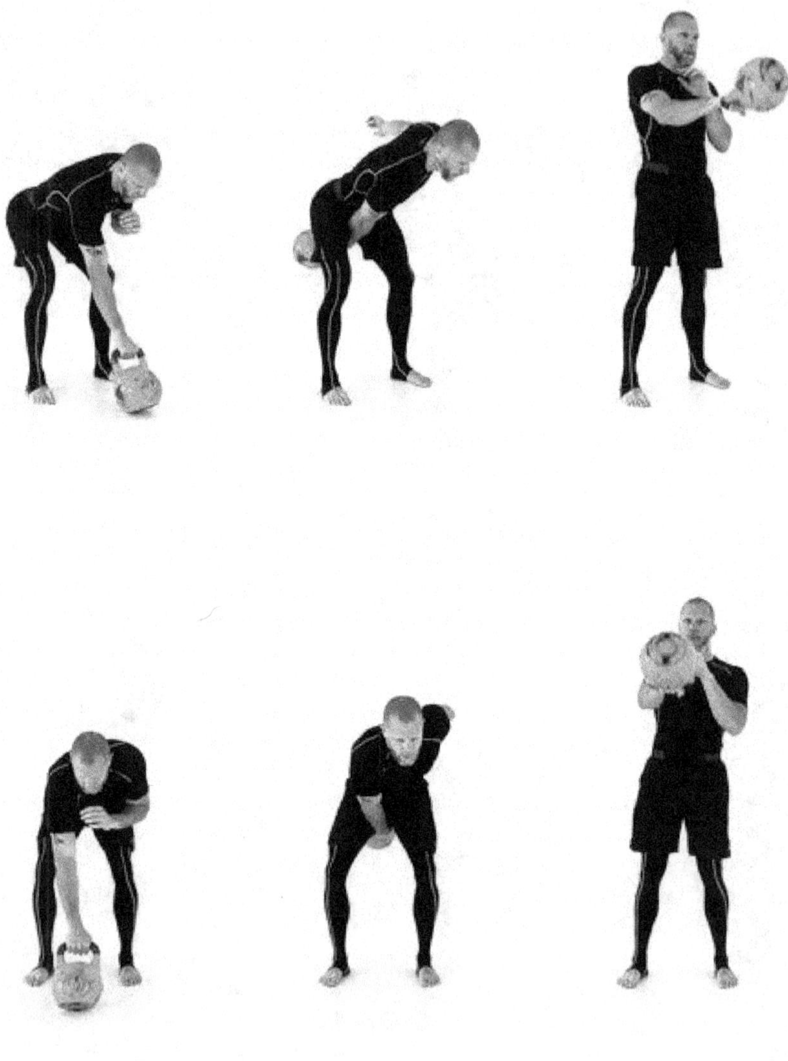

 Kettlebell Exercise Encyclopedia VOL. 4 

## Double Kettlebell

Working with double kettlebells will allow you to work with a lot more load and also remove the rotational pull. One of the things to pay attention to when working with two kettlebells is keeping them together, you do not want a wide gap between them at any stage of the swing.

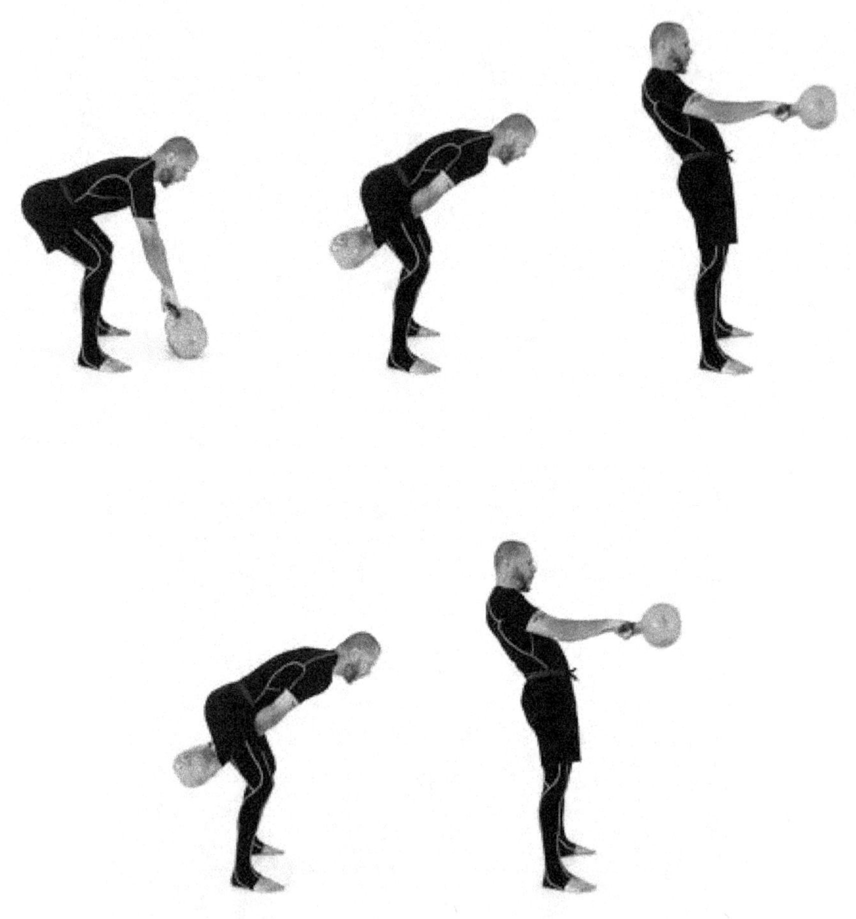

The following two photos display the differences between handle angles. The first photo is a swing with a 90-degree handle angle which turns the thumb up and elbow down.

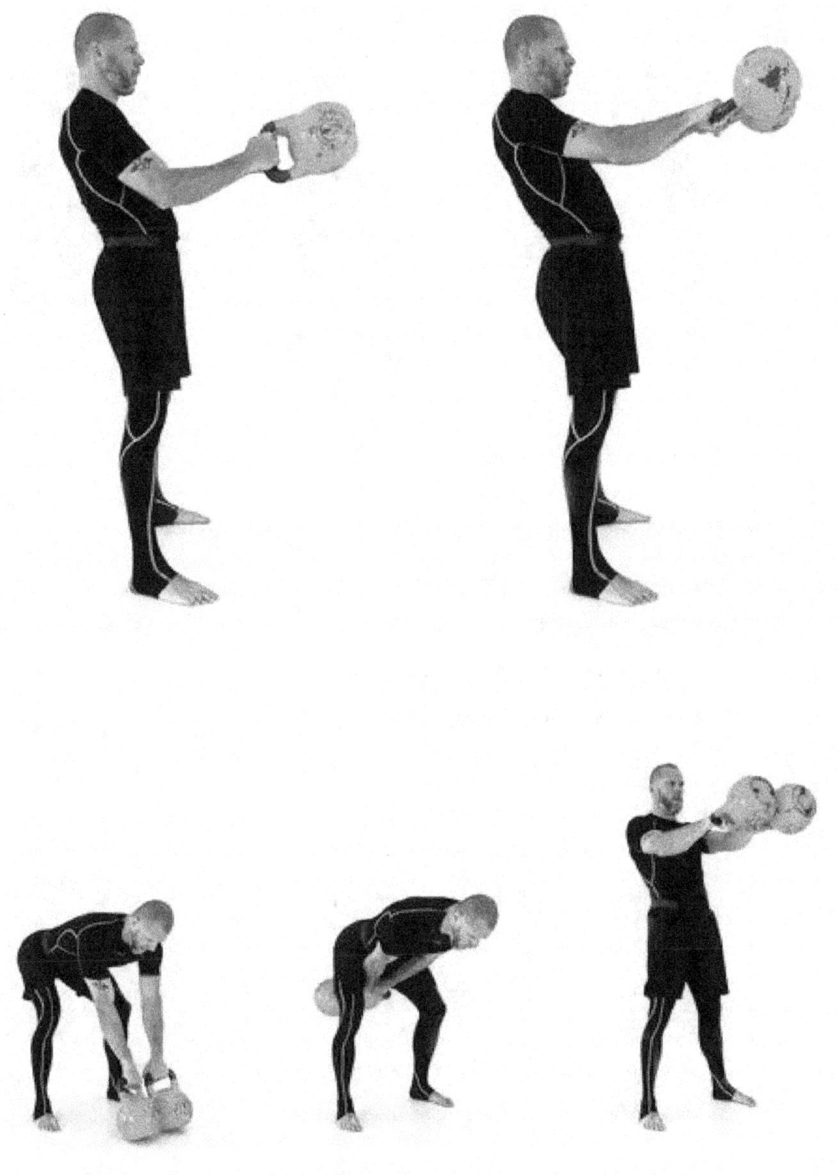

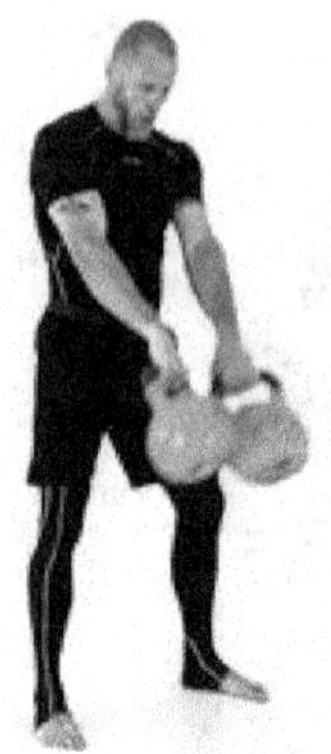 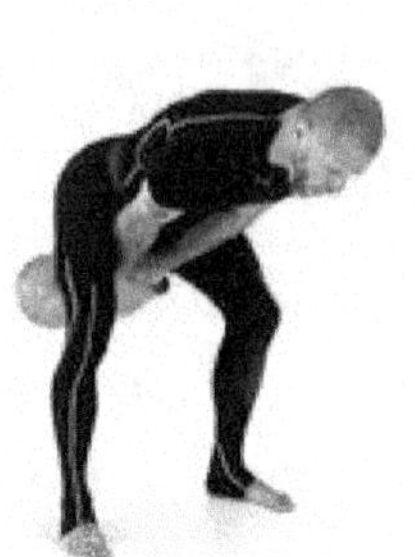 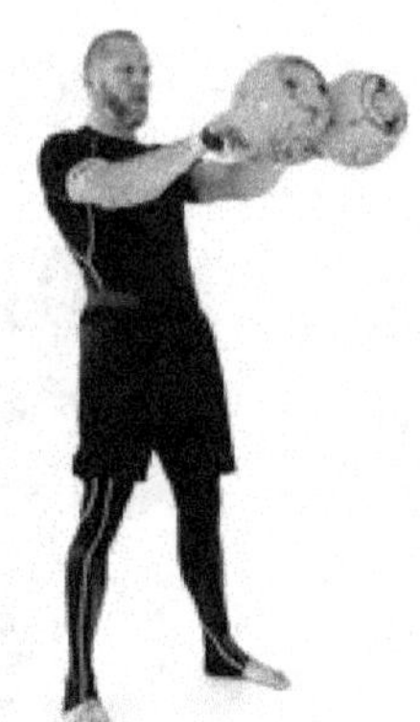

Dot points:

- The hip hinge swing is the most common kettlebell swing

- The movement is wrong when the hip hinge swing is performed with a squat

- Hip hinge and insert

- Pull out and direct the weight forward

- Look ahead at the top of the swing

- Look at the ground in-front at the bottom of the swing

- The hip hinge swing involves two joints for power

- Hips and knees

- The swing can be performed with one joint

- With the hips only it is called the stiff-legged swing

- The swing is going to hurt your back if you do not engage the right muscles intended for the movement

- The right muscles are; gluteus maximus; hamstrings; adductor magnus

- Work on MMC if you experience lower back pain

- Look at technique

- Review programming (reps/weight/rest)

- To protect the lower back you should not follow the kettlebell

- Direct the weight to the back

- Don't let the weight abruptly be stopped by your groin

- Don't let the kettlebell hit your tailbone

- Film and analyze yourself

- Film and ask for a form check
  (reddit.com/r/kettlebell_training, facebook.com/groups/kettebells.for.beginners, or facebook.com/groups/kettlebelltraining)

- The swing can be started with a dead start (dead swing)

- Do low reps when just starting out

- Stop when you have pain and review muscle priming/MMC

- Focus on technique

- You can breathe twice during the swing

- Breathe out at the top and end

- You can breathe once during the swing

- Breathe in on the way down

- Breathe out on the way up

- Don't hold your breath

## Pendulum Swing

The kettlebell sport swing is more about efficiency, removing resistance, going with the flow and it's the foundation for high rep cleans and snatches, i.e. it's specially designed to transition into cleans or snatches, hence it's performed with one arm and one kettlebell. With that said, the fluid style of the sport swing can be applied to double arm one kettlebell as well. The main differences being between this and the conventional swing:

1.  The movement leans more towards quarter squatting and hip hinging

2.  The arms stay connected longer to the body

3.  The movement is powered more by a guided push rather than a pull

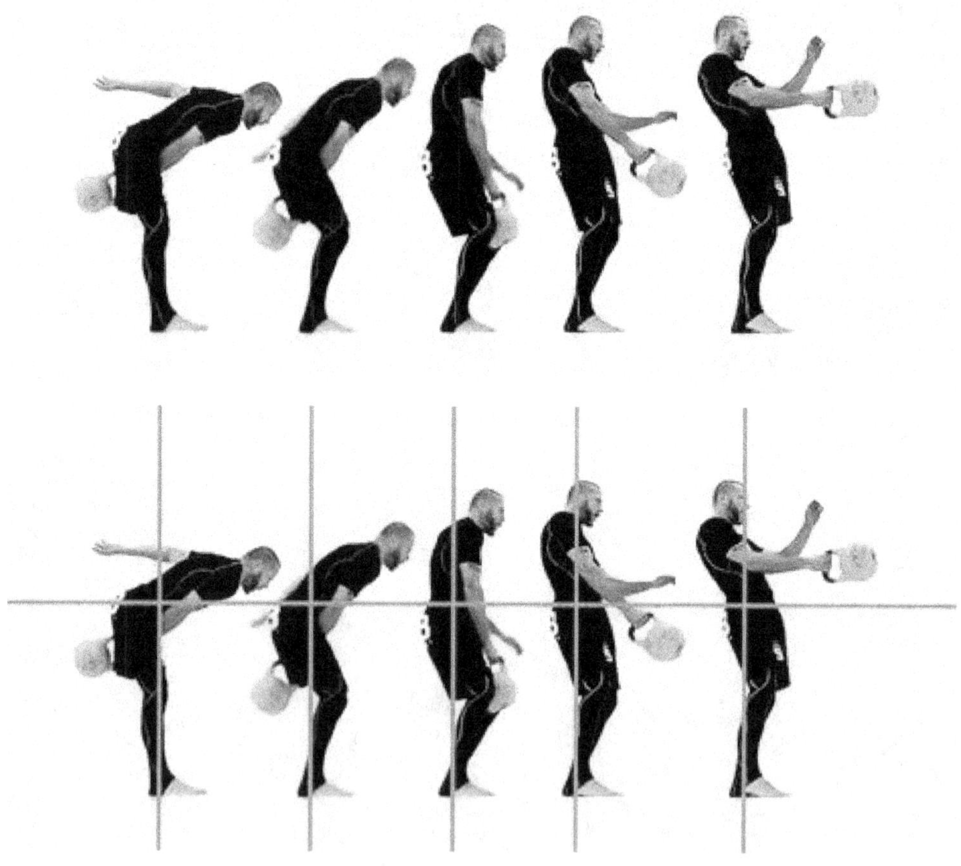

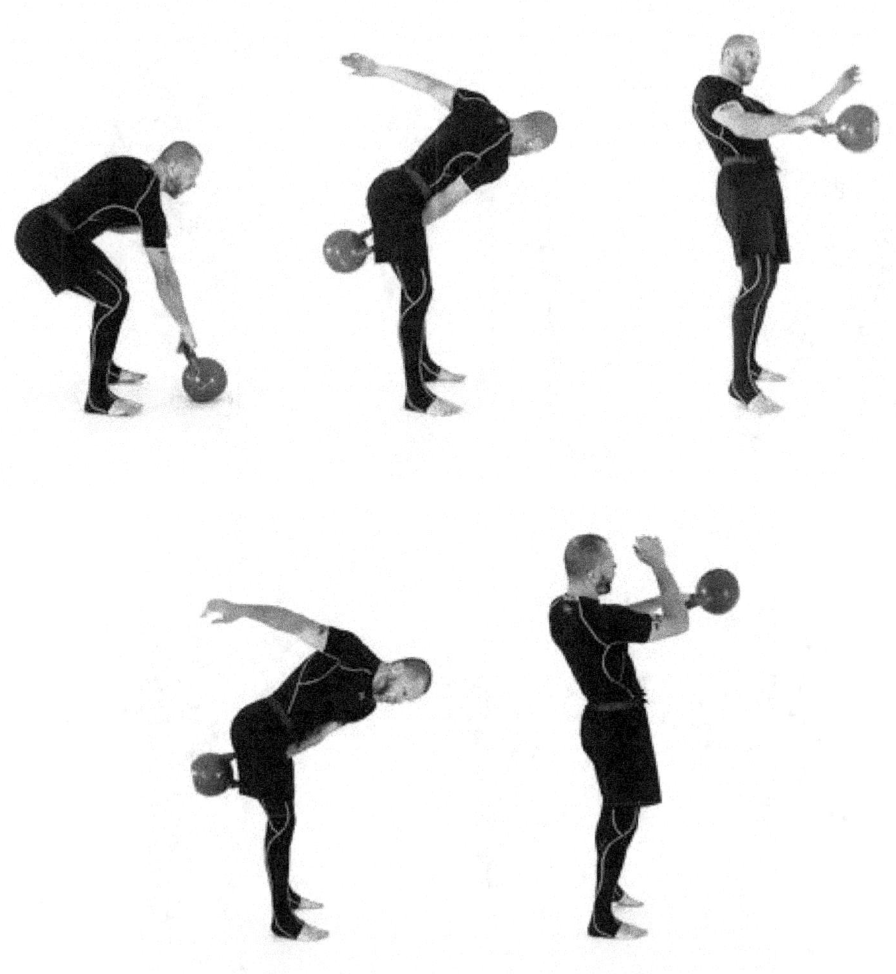

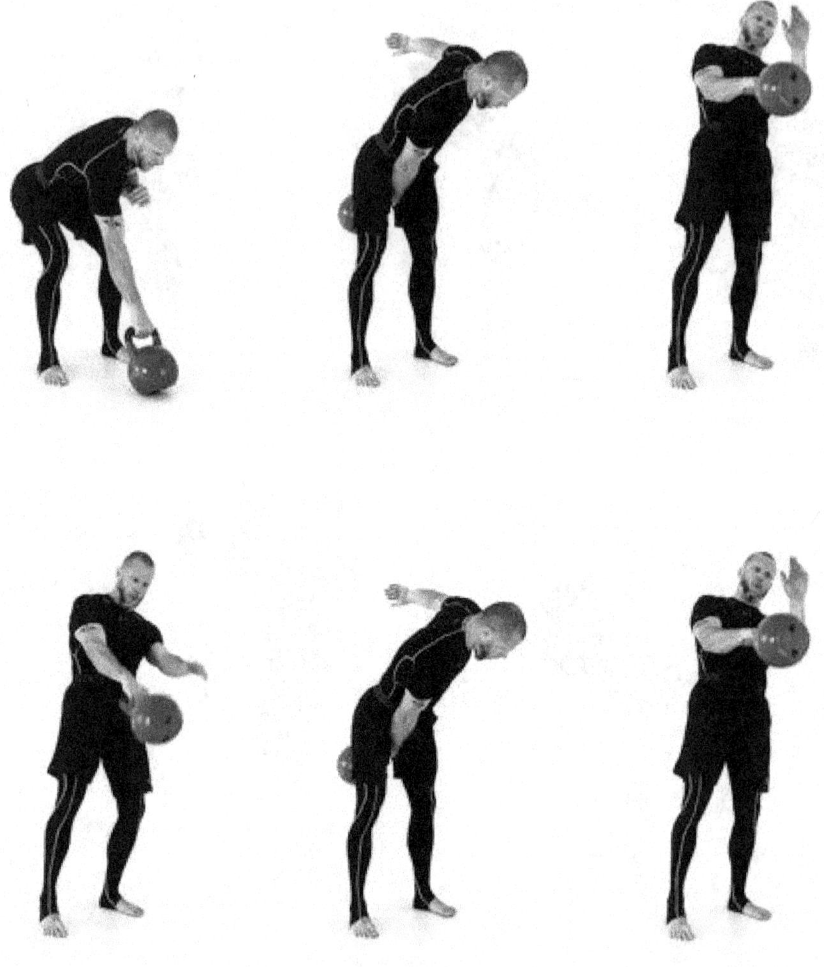

 Kettlebell Exercise Encyclopedia VOL. 4 Taco Fleur

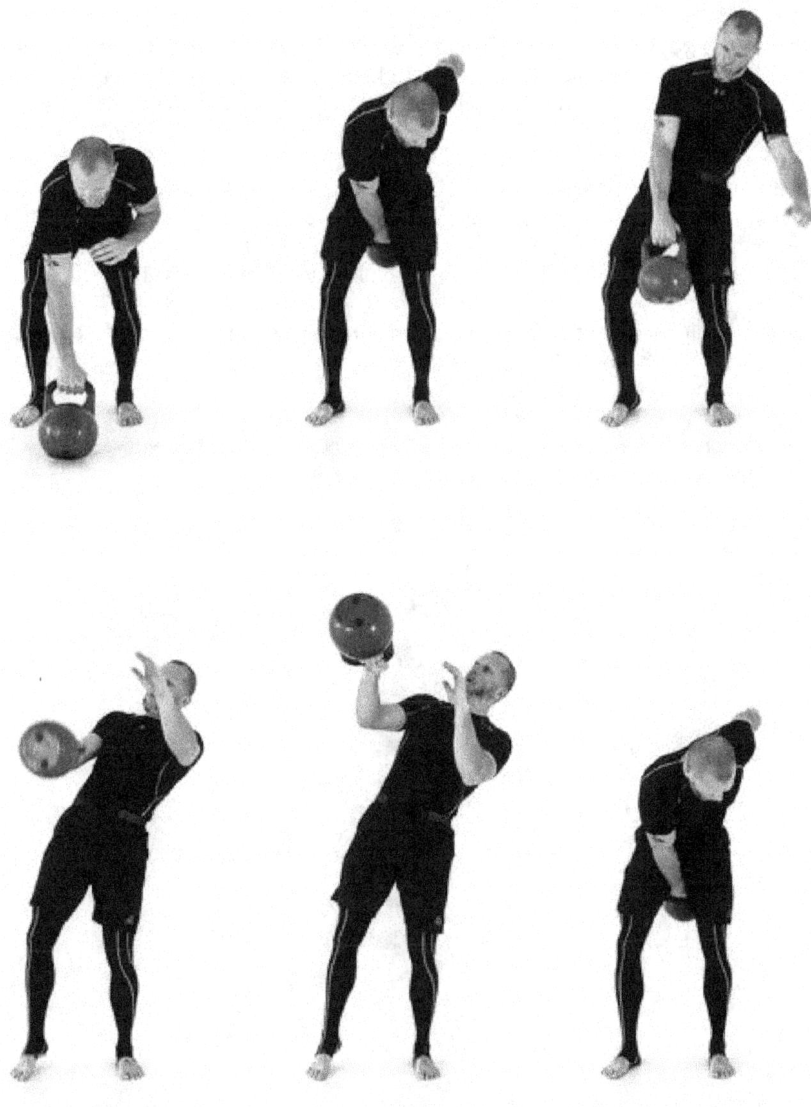

# A pendulum is a weight suspended from a pivot so that it can swing freely.

There are two pendulum concepts in the swing, one relates to your arms, you should never try to shoulder raise the kettlebell during the swing but let them act like a pendulum and move freely. The other is the movement of the swing, it can be a pull or a pendulum, with the first going against resistance, and the second acting upon gravitation and as much as possible like a true pendulum.

It's not a pendulum if your hips are stopping the kettlebell and you're pulling the weight back out, but that doesn't mean it's incorrect, you just need to know when to use one over the other. Do you want to do high or heavy reps or do you want to work your cardiovascular system? Do you want to tax your gluteus maximus as much as possible or do you want to balance it out?

With the pendulum swing, you want to avoid abruptly stopping the kettlebell with your body at the end of the backswing (also cause for bobbing), you can achieve this as best as possible through knee flexion and getting your groin/hips as high as possible. At the endpoint of the backswing, you want to let gravity take control and follow along with the hips to accelerate the weight.

The key is to keep your arms connected to the body as long as possible and push forward while the shoulders are coming up, followed by hip and thoracic hyperextension. When working unilaterally you can also pair this with thoracic rotation.

Your thoracic consists of 12 vertebrae, see Th1 to Th12 below. Together with your cervical this is the area that has the most movement in the spine.

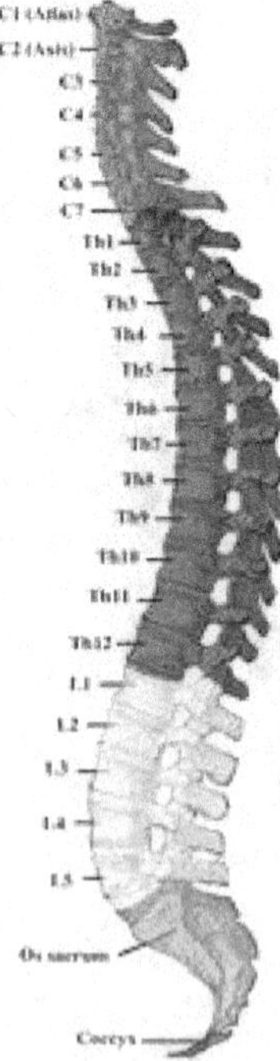

## Pulling versus waiting

There is and always will be some kind of pull happening during the swing, for example, contracting the gluteus maximus, pelvis coming up and the spine following will create a pull through the shoulders coming up, but that all goes to deep in physics. Back to the basics, we're just going to focus on how can you create the most resistance for resistance training, and how can you remove resistance for endurance training.

If you want the most resistance you will create an early pull without waiting till the kettlebell has reached the endpoint of the backswing naturally, and your arms disconnect from the body early, this all provides the most resistance on the gluteals, grip, and other muscles of the posterior chain. If you want the least amount of resistance you will wait for the backswing to naturally end and go along all while increasing velocity. Find a rhythm where gravitation is used with minimum force, in other words, let gravity do as much of the work as possible by adjusting your rhythm.

Not getting your dynamics right could also be cause for friction in the palm, i.e. if you're pulling an object that wants to go the opposite direction will most likely cause handle movement within the palm, which is cause for friction.

## Pull versus push

If you're pulling the kettlebell out and early disconnection happens, the path of the kettlebell is less of an arc and more like a vertical path. How much you're pulling will depend on how fast you come up and how disconnected your arms are. A push of the bell means you're going along with it, your arm(s) remain connected to the body as long as possible. Your knees flex and come forward on the upswing, you're slightly dipping and coming up into full extension.

To perform:
1. Ankles, knees, and hips are extended
2. Kettlebell is at the top of the swing
3. Kettlebell is dropping down into the backswing
4. Depending on how high the swing was, the elbow might be flexed or extended
5. The knees flex paired with ankle dorsiflexion as the weight drops past the hips
6. If the elbow was flexed, it should now be extended
7. The bell is guided on the path of the backswing
8. The hips move back to not stop the weight
9. The knees move into extension paired with ankle plantarflexion
10. The shoulders come toward the ground through hip flexion
11. The weight hits the endpoint of the backswing
12. Gravity takes control and the weight starts falling back
13. The hips follow through with knee flexion paired with ankle dorsiflexion
14. The hips are coming into extension
15. All three leg joints move to full extension
16. The torso is upright
17. The movement should be followed by hip and thoracic hyperextension to create a pull for the snatch
18. The kettlebell moves closer to the body
19. As the bell is closer to the body the elbow needs to bend

20. The weight reaches the point where the magnitude of the velocity is 0
21. The motion of the weight changes ass gravity takes control
22. The weight accelerates downwards and is guided into the backswing for another rep


## Pendulum swing objective

The objective of this swing is to use as much momentum as possible rather than a violent pull. Push along with the weight, and keep the weight close to your body. A bell that's not close to the body will require pulling in or unbalances your posture.

A very important part of the swing is to guide the trajectory up, even though it may look like the kettlebell is pulled in closer through a curl (think biceps curl), this is not the case. The trajectory is created through timing, hip extension, hip hyperextension, thoracic hyperextension, and it can even go paired with thoracic rotation. If you're feeling your elbow flexors (think tendons in the elbow area) then you're actively curling the weight close to the body and your trajectory is off. Doing this multiple times will cause stress on the tendons and can eventually cause tendonitis.

Once more, yes there is elbow flexion, but it's not a curl where the weight is curled in towards the body, the elbow flexion happens by following the trajectory of the kettlebell which is up and close to the body.


## Hip hinge versus pendulum swing

You'll have most likely been swinging a kettlebell already with the hip hinge, which means you're in extension (standing straight) and coming in and out of hip flexion. The main difference between the hip hinge and pendulum swing is that you'll need to perform double extension, once in standing (start and end of swing) and once at the back of the swing. The **extension** happens as follows:

Standing (start and end):

1. hips

2. knees

3. ankles


End of backswing:

1. knees

2. ankles


Back into standing.

The end of the backswing is paired with hip flexion. In between the start, middle, and end, a dip/quarter squat occurs. On the way back this quarter squat moves the hips back, on the way up it moves forward.

1. full extension
2. dip back
3. extension plus hinge
4. dip forward
5. full extension

The dip or quarter squat is:

1. ankle dorsiflexion (which automatically brings the knees forward)
2. knee flexion
3. hip flexion

The movement back is controlled through the extension of three joints.

Dot points:

- There are 3 main movements to perform the swing

- Squat; Hip hinge; Pendulum

- The pendulum swing comes from kettlebell sport

- The pendulum swing is usually performed with one arm

- Make space for the bell

- Stay connected

- Go with the flow

- Don't resist the weight

- This is a push whereas the other two movements are a pull

- Push the arms forward

- Great swing for high volume reps

- Each swing has its own reason for doing them

- The pendulum swing is great for the clean

- There are many different ways to perform the pendulum swing

- The pendulum swing provides the least amount of stress on the body

- Know when to use one over the other

## Squat Swing

The kettlebell swing squat style is performed in a similar fashion to the conventional swing, with the following differences:

1.  Four joints involved rather than three

2.  The upper-body remains more vertical during the swing

3.  The shins no longer remain vertical during the swing and come forward

4.  Ankle dorsiflexion is created

5.  The trajectory of the swing is down and up rather than forward and back

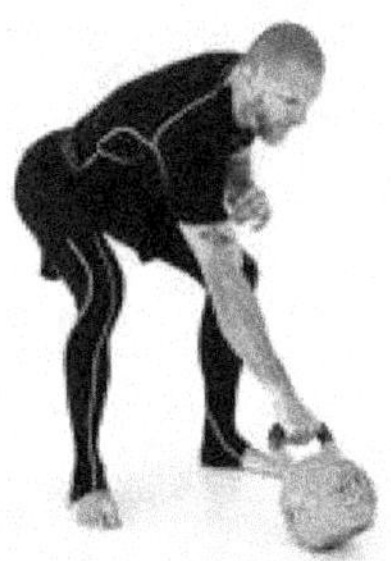 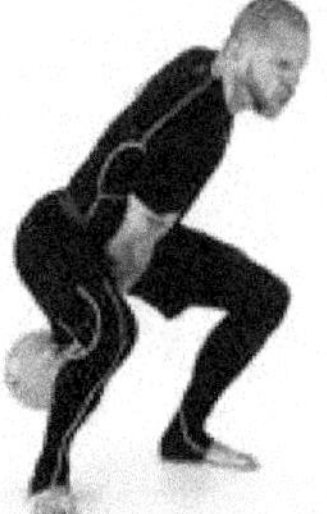 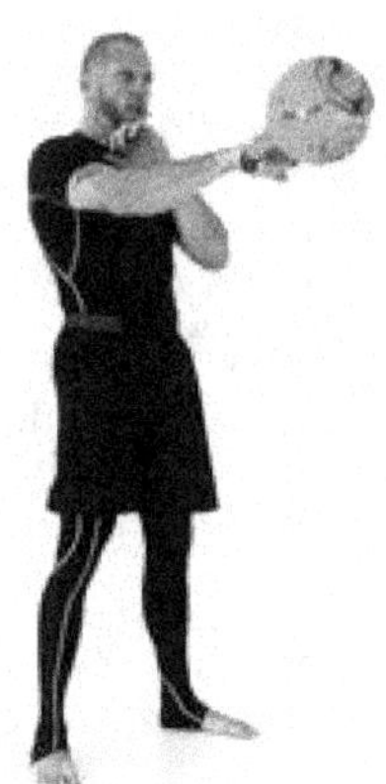

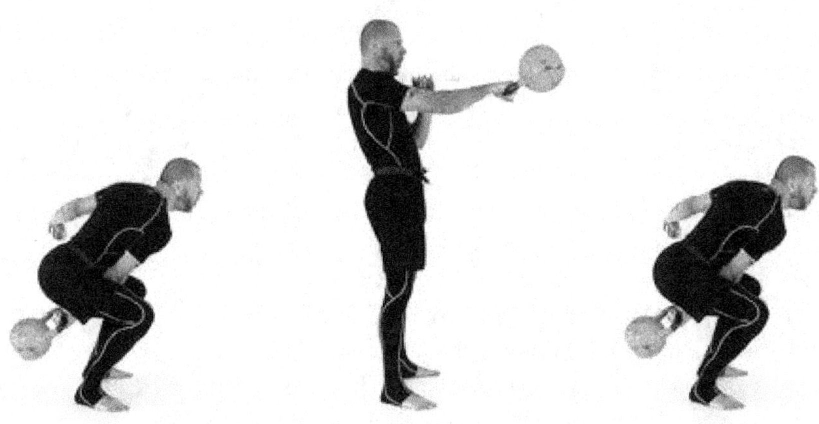

The following two photos display the clear differences between a squat and hip hinge swing. In the first photo, there is clear ankle dorsiflexion (knees coming forward), the hips are lower, and the torso is more upright.

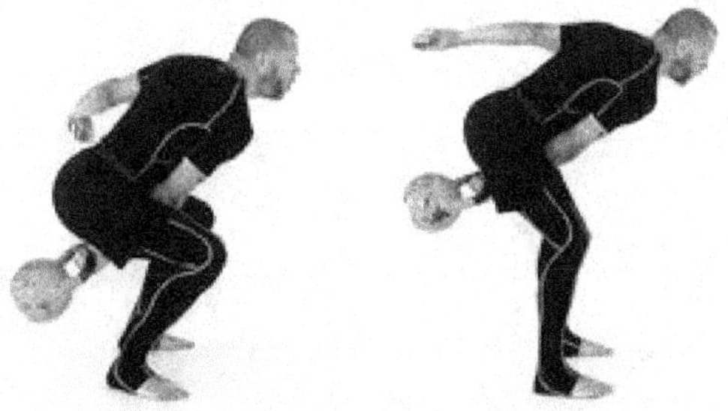

Dot points:

- The kettlebell swing is one of the most popular kettlebell exercises
- There is so much more to kettlebell training than just the swing

- There are many different types of kettlebell swings
- The squat swing is controversial
- A swing is good if it's safe and works towards your goals
- It is important to know why you're doing an exercise
- You should also learn the hip hinge swing
- Understand the differences between the squat and hip hinge
- The squat swing uses more of the anterior muscles and is less stress on the lower back
- The hip hinge is more isolation of the gluteus maximus and provides more stress on the back (not always a bad thing)
- Your arms are just a pendulum with your shoulder being the pivot in the swing
- The only swing that is a shoulder raise is the *American swing*
- Shoulders should be slightly pulled back and down
- Don't pull the kettlebell up with the shoulders
- Drive the weight up with the power from your legs
- To start you bump the weight out and don't worry how high it comes
- If the kettlebell comes too high then the weight is probably too light
- The weight is too heavy if it does not come higher than the hips
- The kettlebell should be a direct extension of your arms at all times
- There should be no bobbing at the end or top of the swing
- If you can see the ground at the bottom of your swing you're probably hip hinging
- You can also start your swing with a dead start (dead swing)
- You need more flexibility for the dead start
- Don't overreach for the kettlebell
- Whether you keep your arms straight or bent depends on the trajectory of the kettlebell
- If the kettlebell trajectory is away from you then the arms should remain straight
- If the kettlebell trajectory is up then you can bend your arms
- Guiding the kettlebell away from you adds more back muscle recruitment
- Bent arm with the trajectory being out and away creates tension/tugs on the elbow flexors

## Single Kettlebell Double Arm

1. Bump the weight out to start
2. Let the weight freely dropdown
3. Guide the weight between the legs and towards the ground
4. Bend the three joints for the squat
5. Keep the shoulders high
6. Look ahead
7. Pull the weight back up
8. Come back upright
9. Push the heels into the ground
10. Pull the knees back

11.Extend the hips
12.Let the weight come up and forward
13.Come into full extension
14.The weight reaches about chest height
15.Let the weight drop back down
16.Repeat

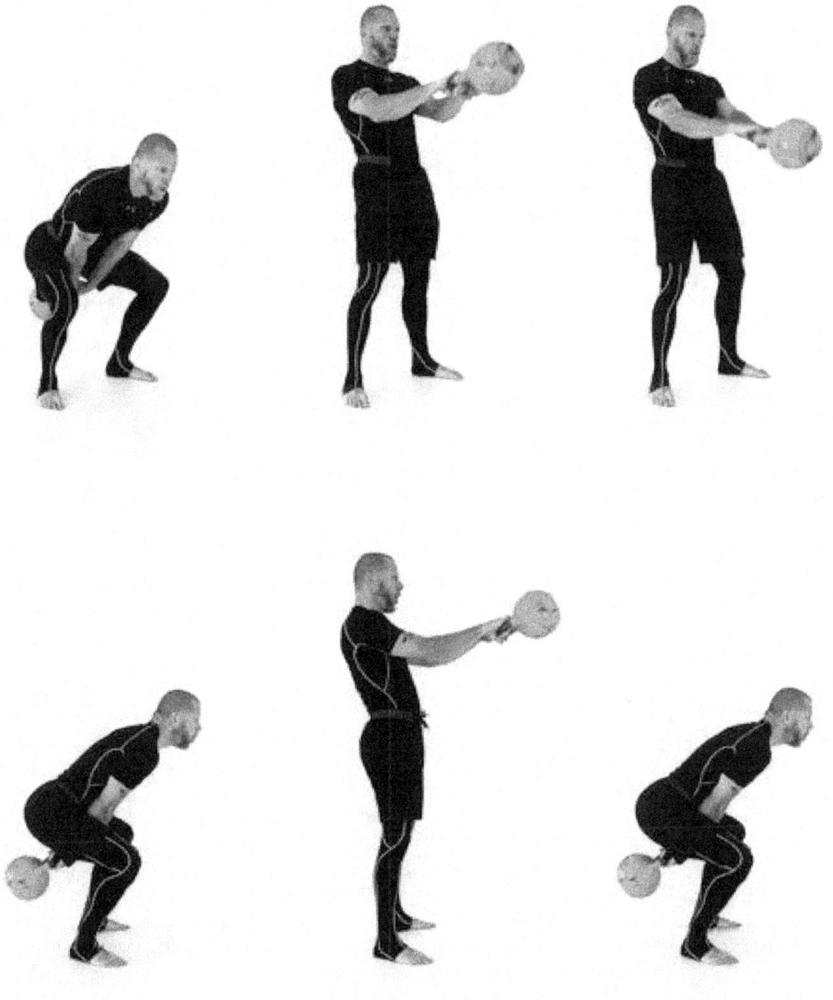

# Suitcase Swing

AKA: Side swing

Variations:
- Single-arm one kettlebell
- Double-arm two kettlebells

The suitcase swing is commonly performed hip hinge style, but the heavier the kettlebell, the more it will lean towards squat style. This swing is different from the common swings due to the kettlebell(s) swinging on the outside rather than through the legs.

1. More lat activation required

2. Feet are closer together to allow the kettlebell(s) to swing on the outside

3. Thumb can be pointing inwards or upwards which dictates the angle of the handle during the swing

4. More power required to perform the movement

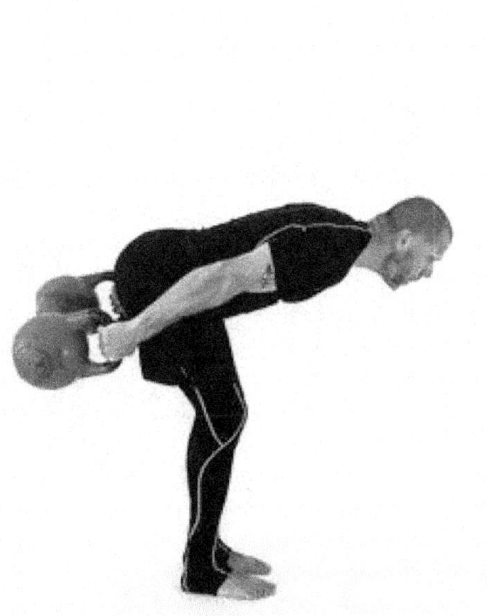

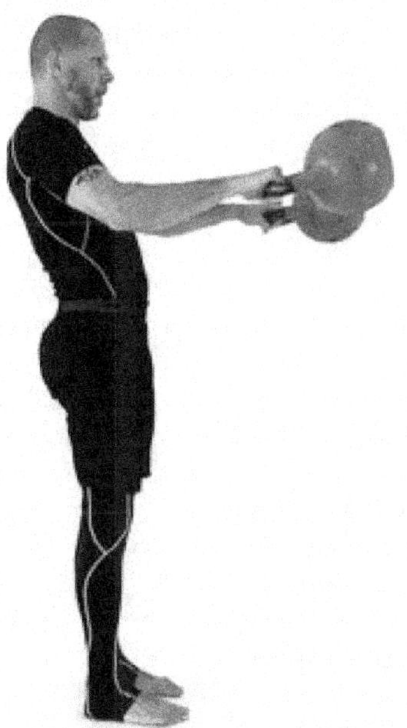

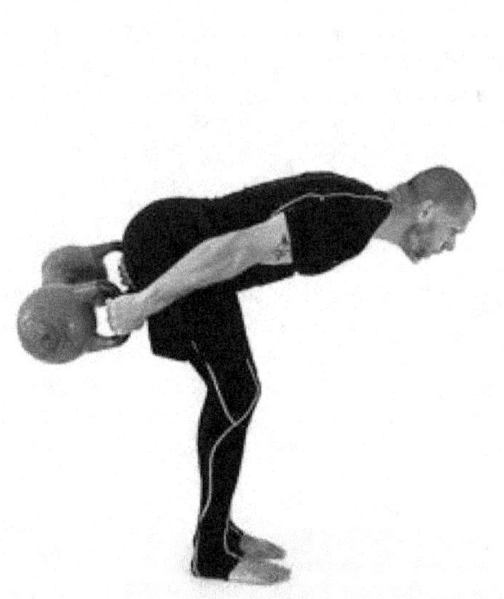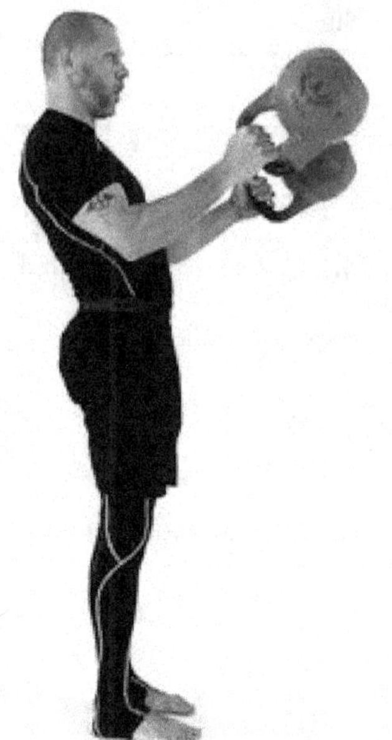

# Swing High Pull

*Combo*

Variations:
- Single-arm one kettlebell
- Double-arm two kettlebells

This swing adds an additional pull to the exercise which is performed high. You can build this upon several different swing variations, see conventional, squat, or pendulum swing.

To perform:

1. Perform a swing

2. During the upswing pull the elbow back

3. Squeeze the shoulder blades slightly together

4. The kettlebell should end up about eye level

5. As the kettlebell falls back down you push it out

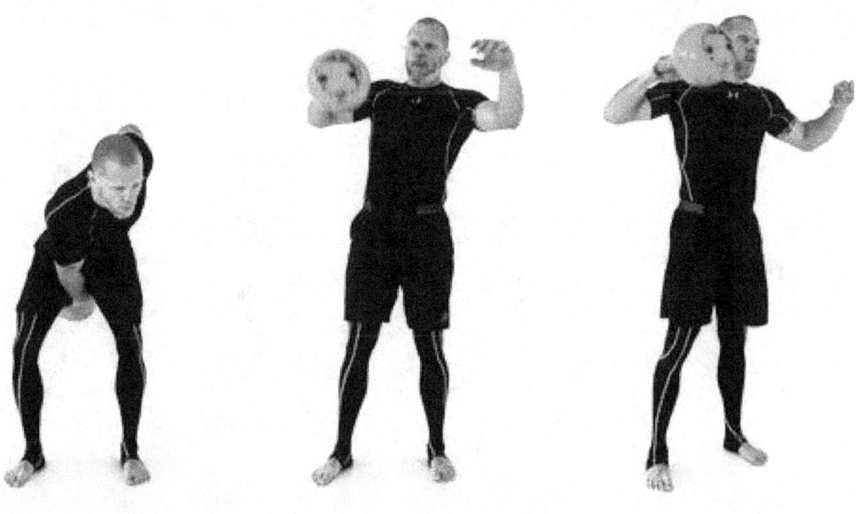

## Short Lever Swing

The short lever swing is a variation of the swing where the elbows bend upon each rep and the kettlebell is positioned close to the chest at the top of the swing. The short lever swing can be used as the first half of the American swing, and with enough power the kettlebell comes higher and is then pressed out.

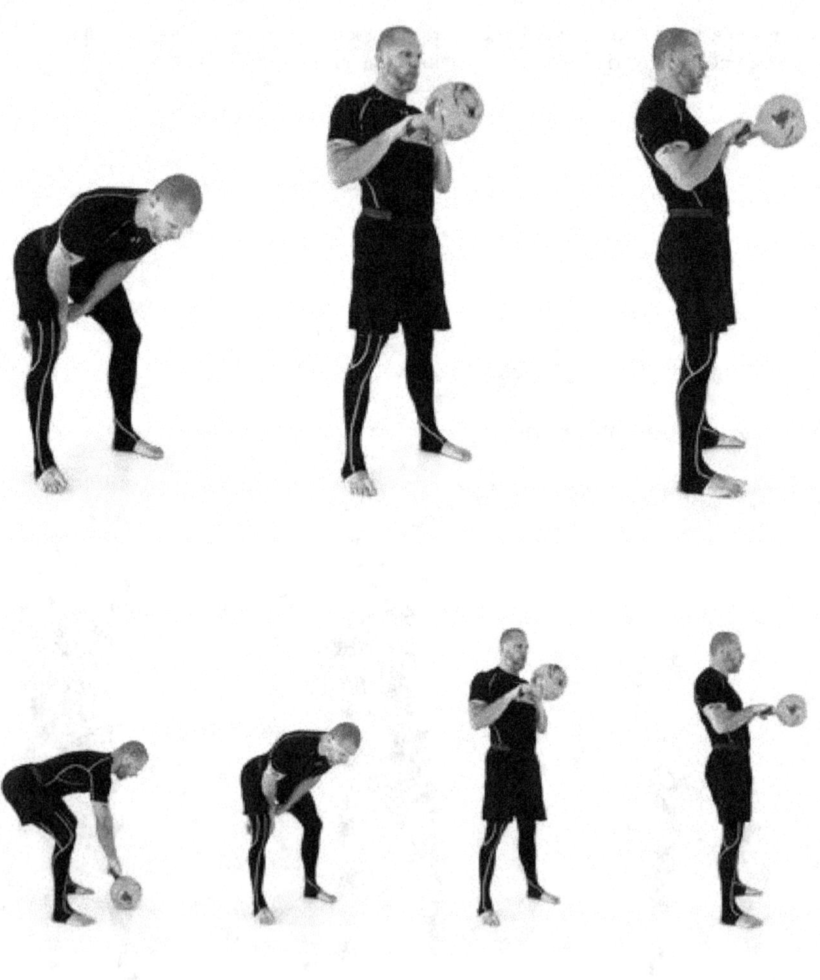

## Side-Step Swing

Variations:
- Double arm one kettlebell

The side step swing is commonly performed with the hip hinge style swing, the difference being:

1. You're moving laterally by stepping sideways to the left or right upon each upswing

2. Your legs are close together at the top of the swing

3. You're stepping sideways on the down-phase of the swing


## Walking Swing

Variations:
- Single-arm one kettlebell
- Double-arm one kettlebell
- Double-arm two kettlebells

With this swing, you're either moving forward or backward and is great for coordination, commonly performed hip hinge style. Everything from the conventional swing applies with the added difference that on the up-phase of the swing you're following through and stepping forward or backward.


## Lateral Swing

Variations:
- ! Single-arm one kettlebell
- ! Double-arm one kettlebell

Targets: Core, obliques, rotatores, rotational

This is a rotational exercise and great for golf, baseball, boxers or other martial arts as it targets the obliques. There is no hip hinge or squat in this swing, all the power is generated through the rotation of the spine.

To perform:

1. Feet hip-width apart and slightly turned outwards

2. Hold the kettlebell with two hands

3.  Elbows always extended

4.  Let the kettlebell hang on one side of the body

5.  Rotate into the side where the kettlebell hangs

6.  Rotate to the other side

7.  Pivot on the foot that's away from the kettlebell

8.  Generate enough power to get the kettlebell to lateral shoulder height

9.  Guide the kettlebell back down and shift the hips to the other side

10. Pivot the other foot

11. Rotate the thoracic spine

12. And drive the hips through to get the kettlebell up to shoulder height on the other side

13. Eyes follow the kettlebell

14. Think of this as three positions:

    ○ Kettlebell positioned laterally on one side about shoulder height with the foot on the other side pivoting

    ○ A neutral front-on position where the bell is swinging past the knees

    ○ Kettlebell positioned laterally on the other side about shoulder height with the foot on the opposite side pivoting

It's completely opposite to the conventional swing where in neutral front-on position the kettlebell would be shoulder height, with this swing it's positioned and swinging past the knees going upward laterally.


## Power Swing

The power swing is a swing performed with the hip hinge movement and the part that makes this a power swing is the speed at which you perform this. Not only do you explode up but you also explode down, you're actively pulling/pushing the kettlebell down into the backswing. This is also a great swing to do with a partner, i.e. you swing and your partner pushes the kettlebell back down with force.

## Dead Swing

Variations:

>   ! Single-arm one kettlebell
>   ! Double-arm one kettlebell
>   ! Double-arm two kettlebells

This variation of the swing can be performed in any style. The kettlebell needs to return dead to the ground upon each rep which is great for working on explosiveness with heavyweights. The description of the movement is as easy as combining the hike back and conventional or another style swing.

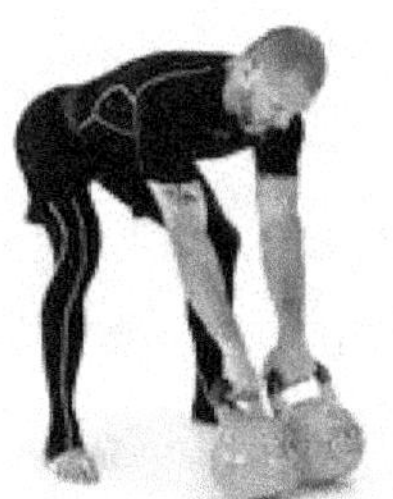 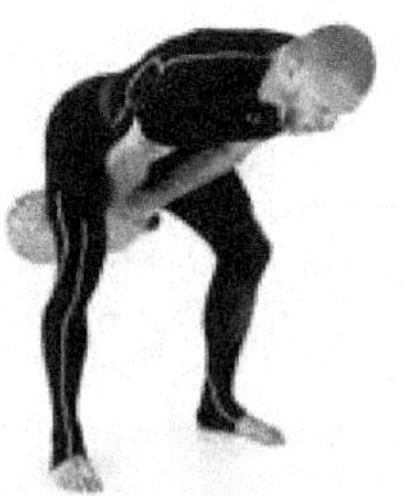 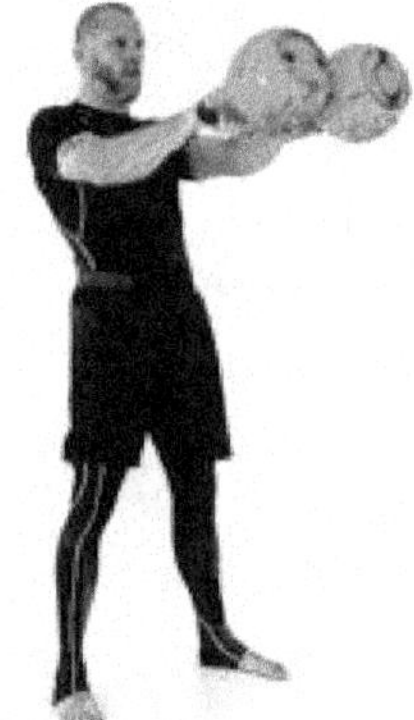

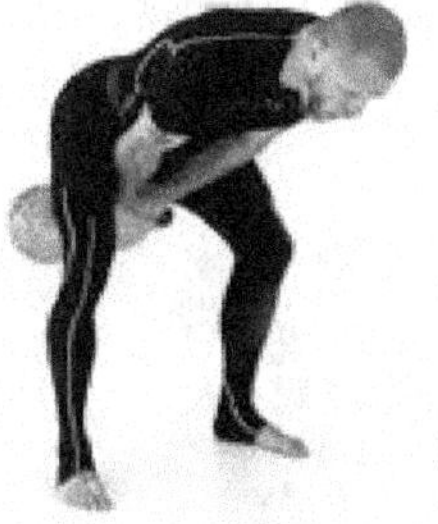 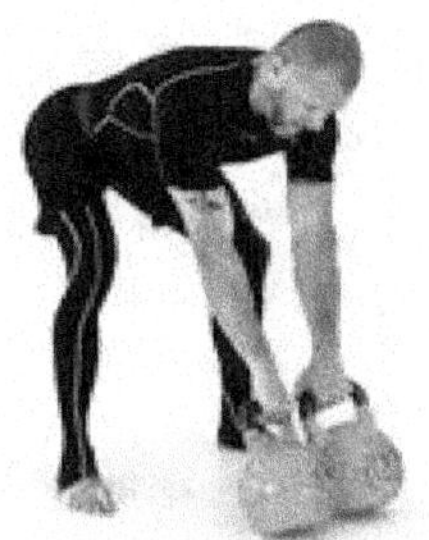



Kettlebell Exercise Encyclopedia VOL. 4

# Kettlebell Windmill

The windmill is an exercise where the torso comes laterally to the side and forward (hinge) while both legs remain straight or one slightly bend. The movement is paired with thoracic rotation and one arm overhead while the other reaches for the ground or opposite foot. The benefits of this exercise are core strength, thoracic rotation, shoulder strength, shoulder rotation, and a good stretch in the hamstrings.

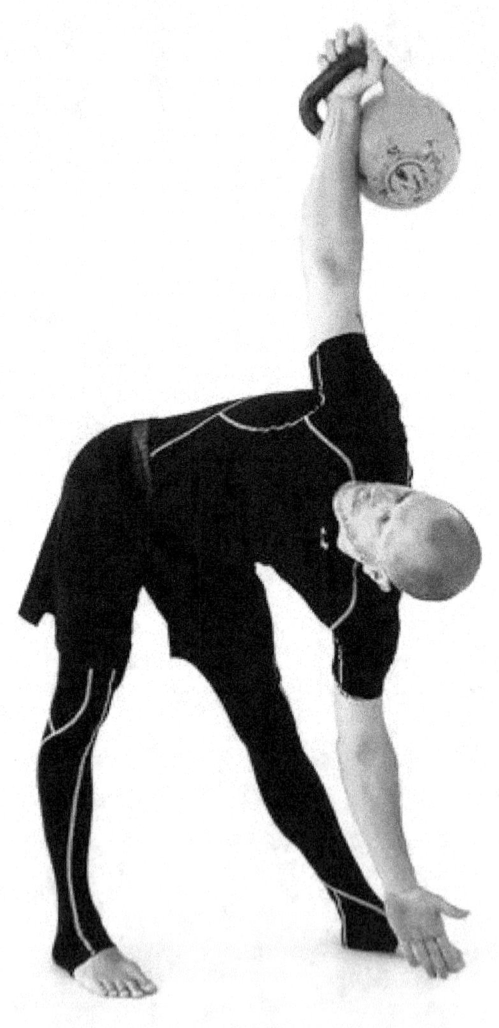

# Kettlebell High Windmill

The high windmill is just like the bodyweight windmill with the obvious difference being it is loaded with a kettlebell. You'll require more shoulder stability and work in the obliques and quadratus lumborum. The added weight will also work the strength of the triceps to keep the arm straight (elbow locked out). The additional stability required will obviously trickle down, shoulders, spine, hips, etc.

In the photos, you'll see that you can reach for your opposite foot or the foot directly under you. Whatever you do, don't force the range and just let progression happen naturally.

Before you attempt the kettlebell windmill you should master the movement without weight. You're getting a good stretch in the hamstrings of the straight leg, obliques, and thoracic. You're also getting shoulder rotation in the arm at the top. As you can see, many benefits from just one exercise.

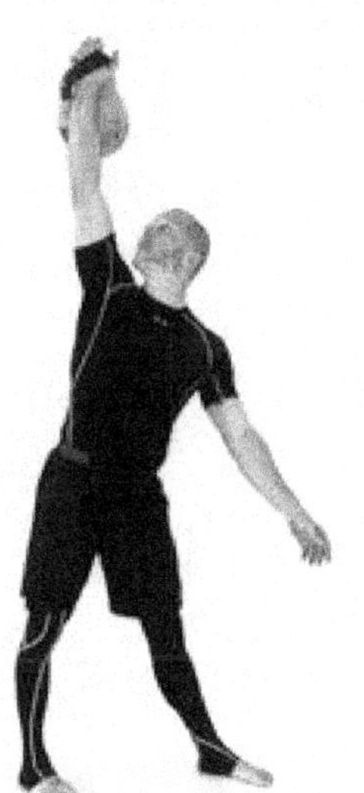 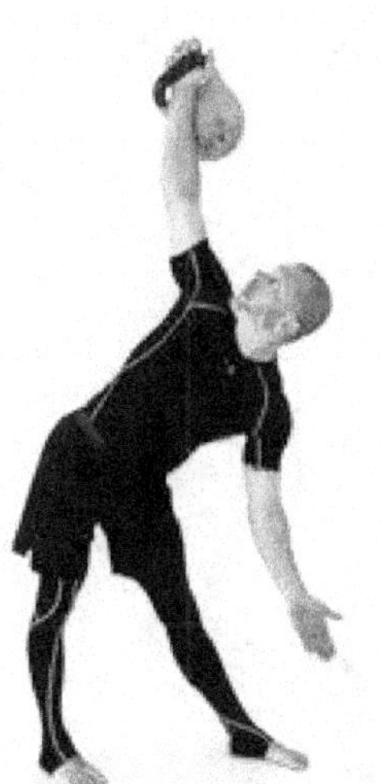 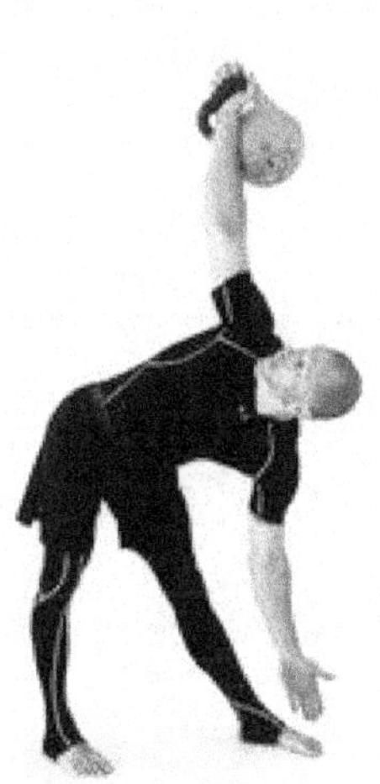

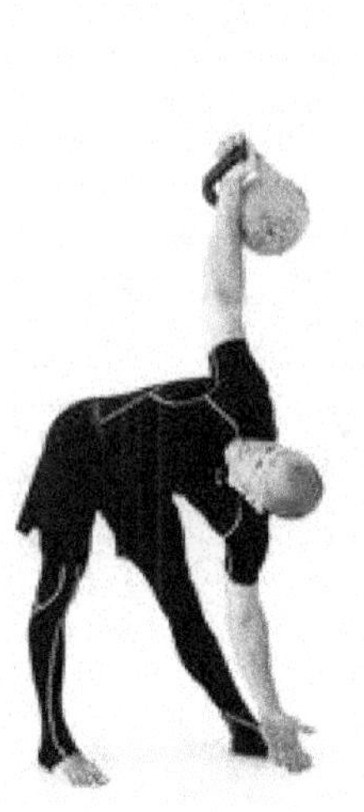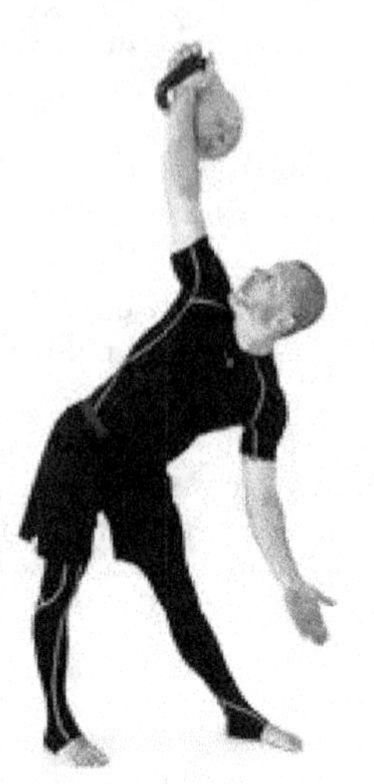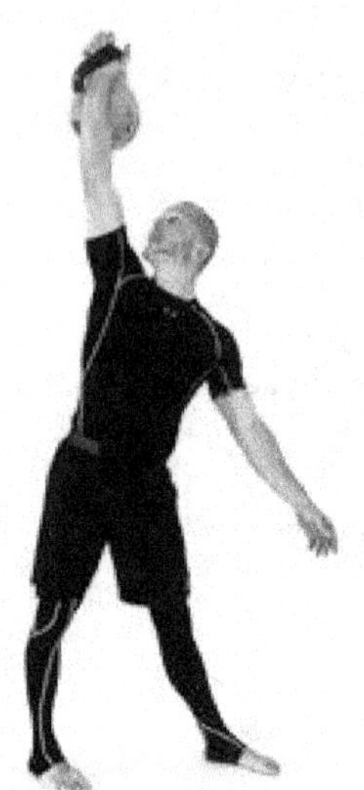

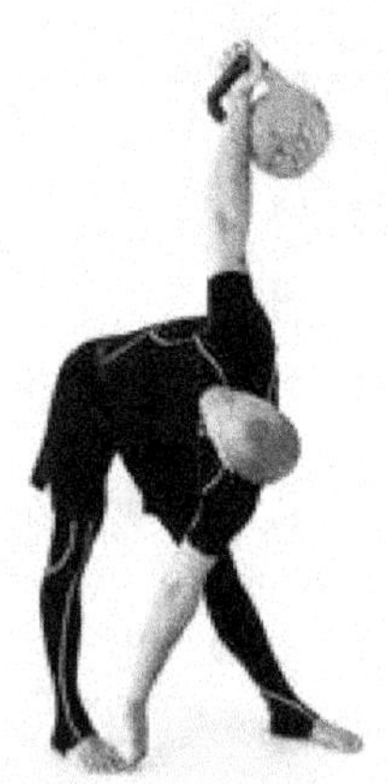

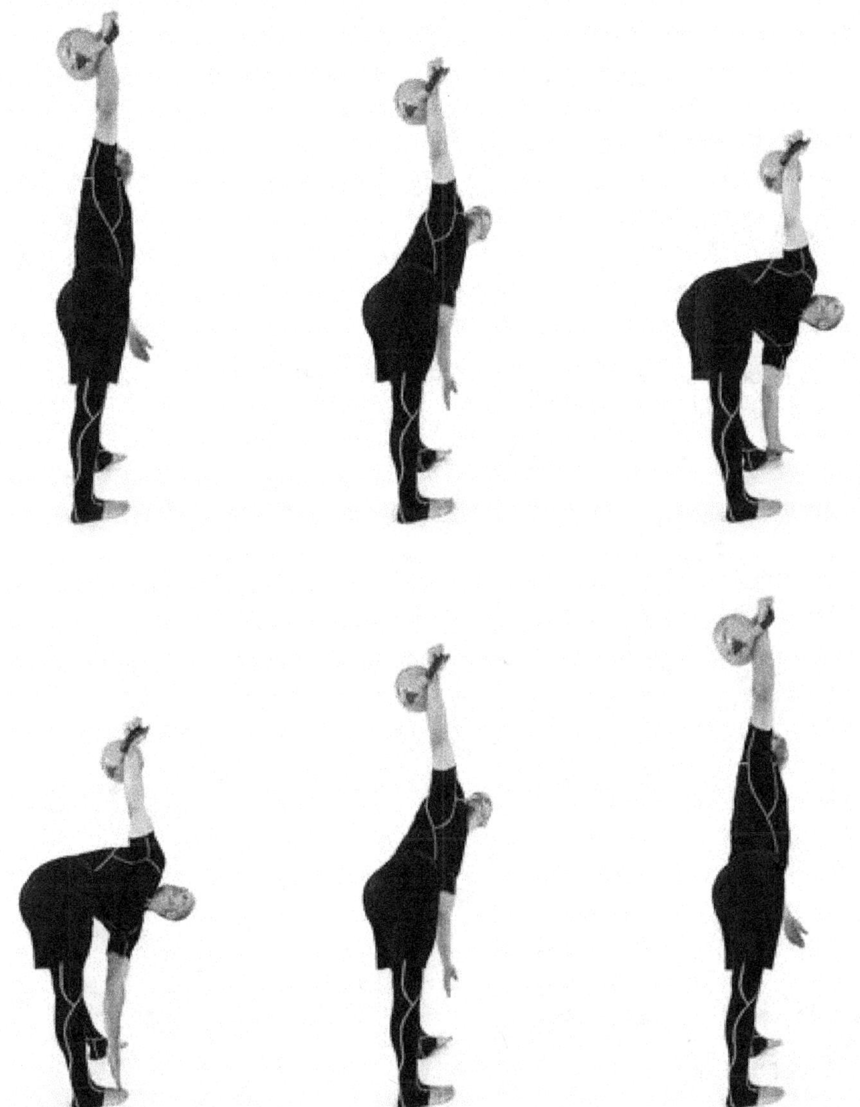

**To perform:**

- Stand in a neutral stance

- Decide which side you're going to perform the windmill in

- Raise the arm on the side you'll be moving away from

- The leg stays vertical on the side you're moving away from

- Step out laterally into the side you will be performing the windmill in

- The foot should be approximately at a 45-degree angle

- Slightly adjust the angle of the foot on the vertical leg turning inward

- With the diagonal leg push the hip into and above the vertical leg

- Keep pushing throughout the down phase of the movement

- Keep the spine straight

- Bend at the hips and come to the side

- Keep your head neutrally aligned with the spine

- Create thoracic rotation as you're coming down through pulling the bottom shoulder forward and the top shoulder back

- Slight shoulder rotation as you're moving down

- Move with the intention to put the hand of the bottom arm to the floor near your foot

- Reach maximum range without bending the spine

- Feel the stretch in the hamstrings of the vertical leg

- Come back up by activation of the quadratus lumborum and obliques located on the side of the vertical leg

Repeat or alternate, when alternating make sure to adjust the angle of the feet and raising the other arm.

If you would bend at the hips coming straight forward and then pushing one hip forward while pulling the other back you would end up in the same position. You should experience this to get a true understanding of the bottom position of the movement.

**Benefits:**

- Shoulders

- Hamstring stretch

- Stability

# Kettlebell Low Windmill

The low windmill is where the kettlebell is lifted from the ground upon each rep or from a hang, depending on flexibility. Although this might sound like an easy progression to the high windmill, it's actually more difficult to lift the weight from the ground than it is to keep it high. The low windmill is a progression to the anyhow windmill.

## Windmill Anyhow

The anyhow windmill is one of the most challenging variations of the windmill when it comes to strength. You'll be working with two kettlebells, one will be overhead while you curl the bottom kettlebell. Before you curl the weight you will need to create a super solid and rigid base to curl with. Progress with a super lightweight on the bottom and super slow movement, make sure you have your breathing and internal pressure under control before attempting this exercise.

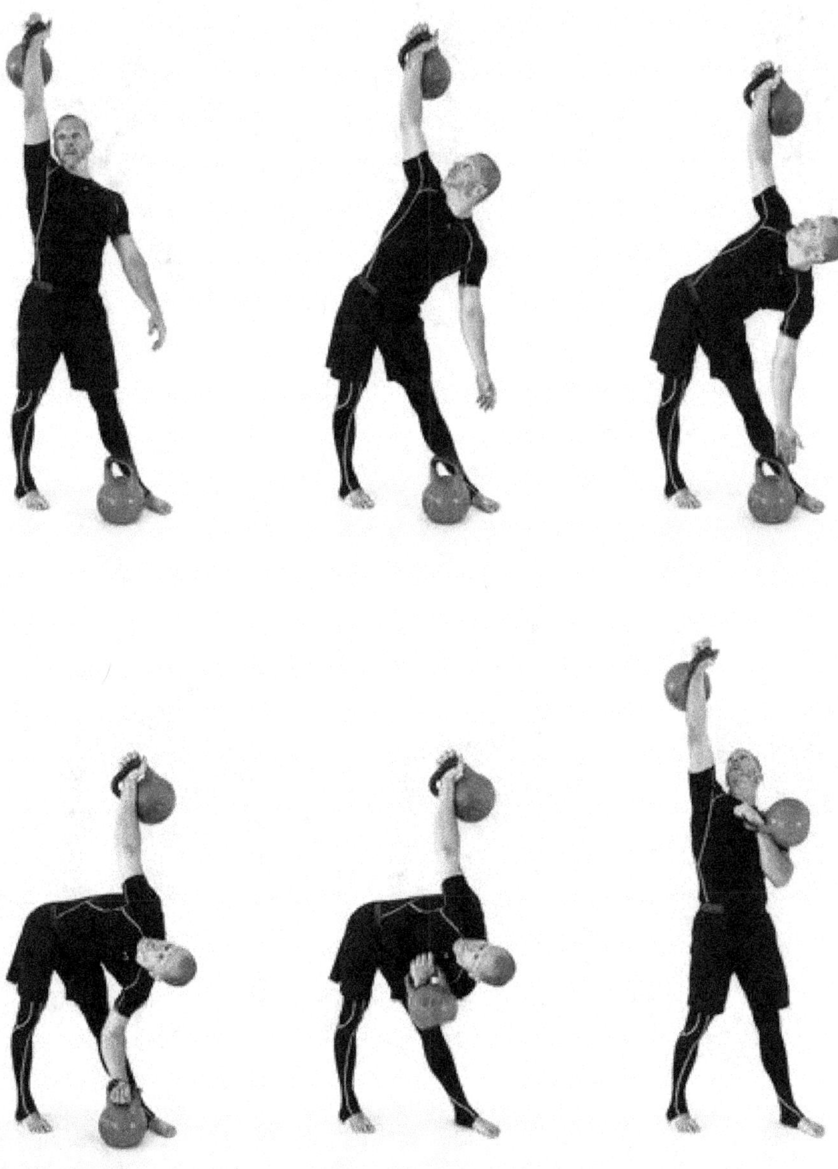

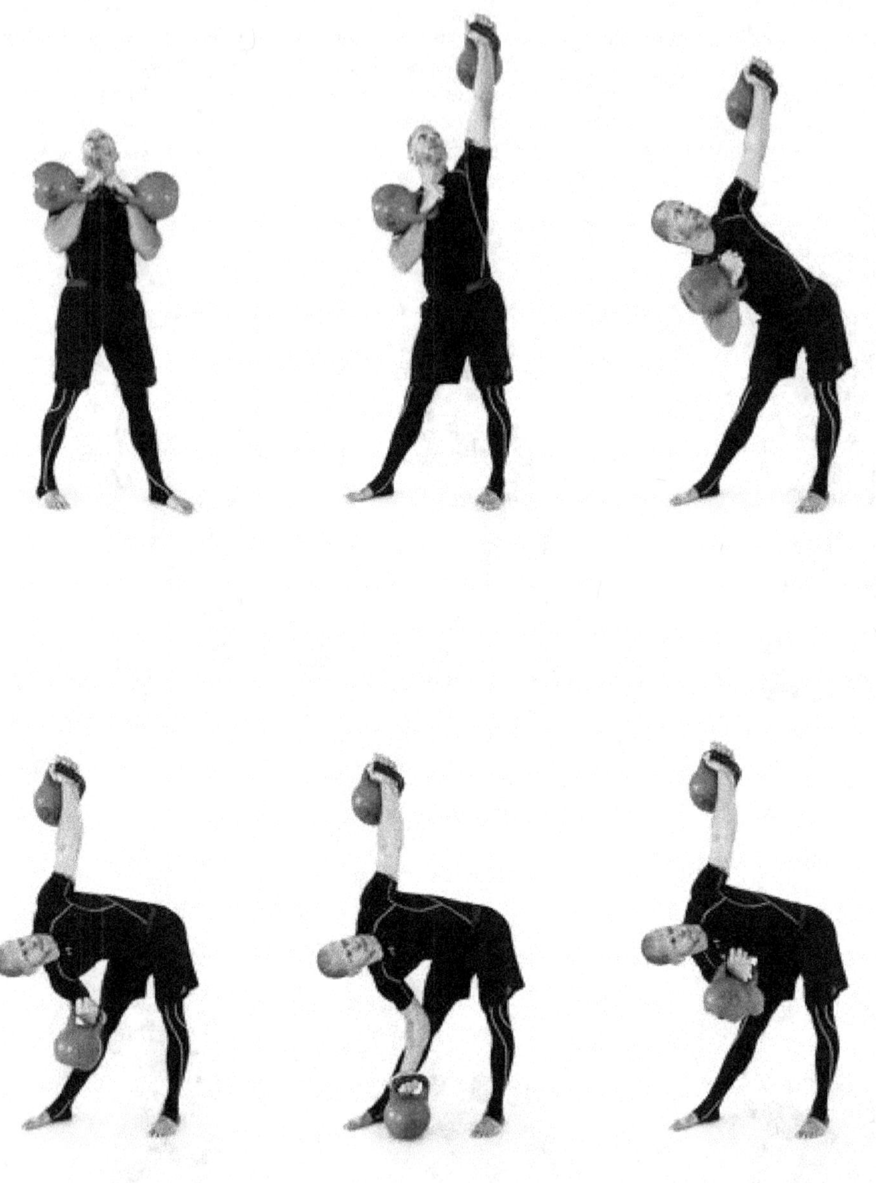

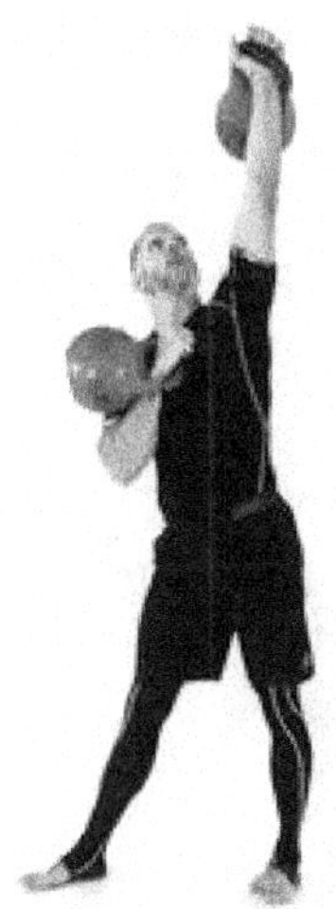

Resting the elbow somewhere on the leg for support will make the curl easier.

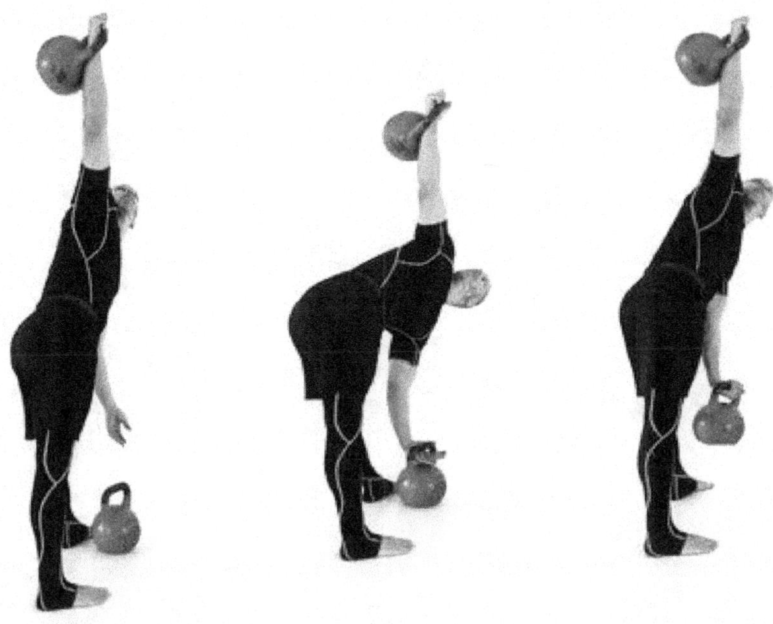

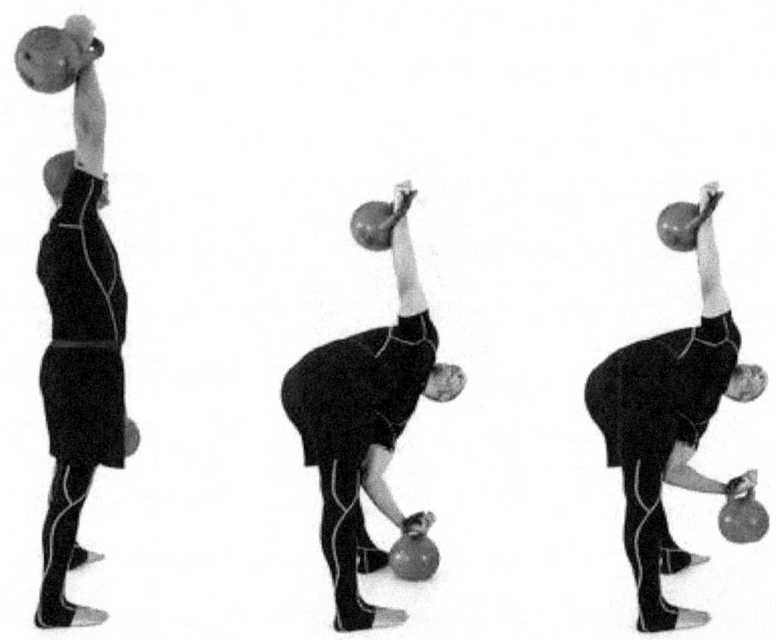

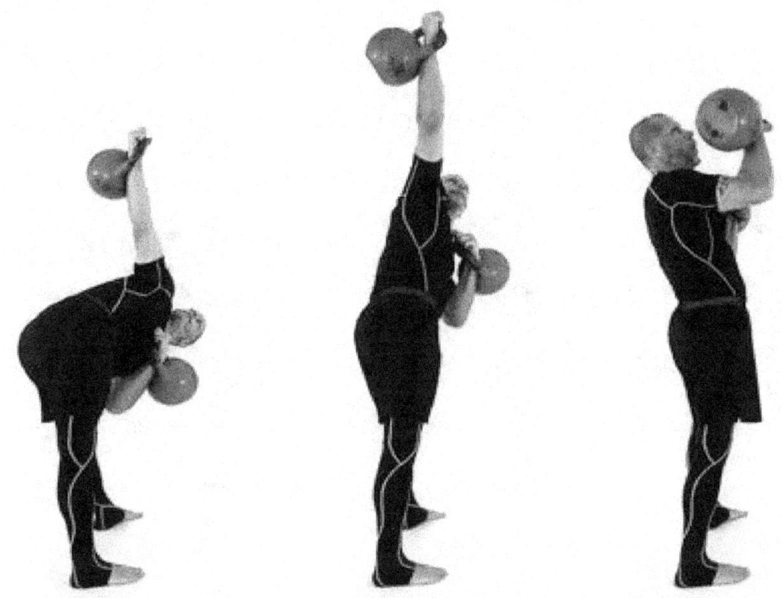

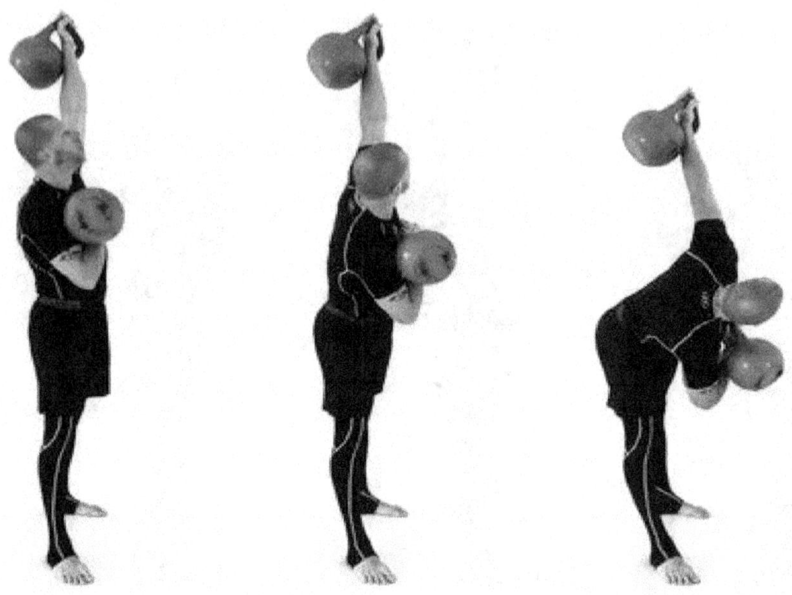

Before you perform the curl make sure to contract everything to create a solid base to curl from.

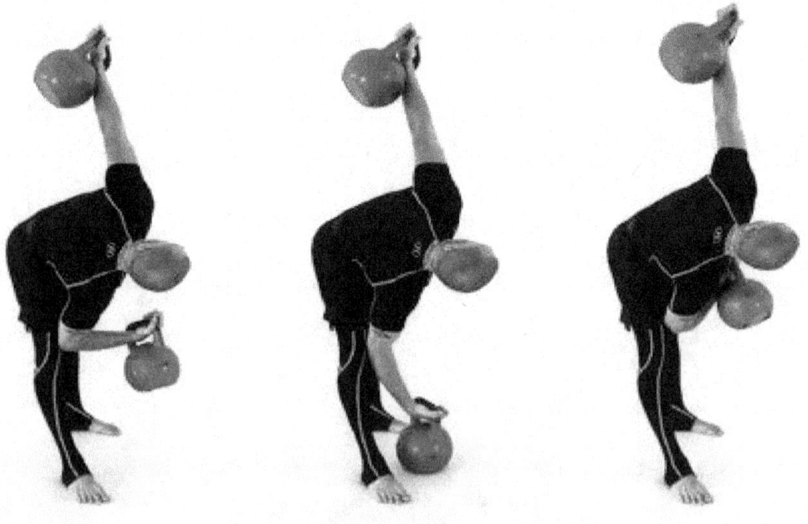

## 90/90 Windmill

I designed this variation of the windmill in 2019 for the *Cavemantraining* program CAVEMANROM.

- 90/90 position (one side hip lateral rotation and other hip medial rotation)
- Bell positioned on the side where the knee is pointing the furthest away
- Come forward at the hips and keep the spine straight
- Curl the weight
- Come back up by pushing the leg into the ground (hip abduction paired with hip lateral rotation)
- Press or bent press (press or come under while pressing)
- Lower to the ground
- Keep sliding the arm out
- Armpit to the knee
- Stabilize the shoulder throughout the movement
- Stay in the bottom position for a second or so and feel the back do work
- Press the leg into the ground (contract the gluteals for hip abduction paired with hip lateral rotation)
- Feel the gluteals doing the work on the side you're pushing away from
- Come back up straight into 90/90 position
- Come forward to lower the weight to the ground
- Come back up and repeat

I failed to get photos for this exercise in time but wanted to include it, I do have a video available: go.cavemantraining.com/kbe-vid-131

# Kettlebell Kneeling Windmill

The benefit of a kneeling windmill versus a standing windmill is that you'll take out the ankles and knee joints, this you will feel in the hip extensors of the kneeling side, and in the hamstrings on the lunging side, more work needs to be done if you're correctly working on balance and posture. You'll be lower to the ground so you won't be able to go as deep which makes it a good progression to the standing windmill, assuming the strength in the lower body is there.

At the bottom of the windmill, you can place your hand on the ground or you can go deeper by bending the elbow and bringing the forearm to the ground. Again, a progress that can be used to progress with depth.

Another great variation that can be used is going from the bottom of the windmill into the runner's lunge by lifting the rear knee off the ground. Doing so will work the lats on the side the hand/arm is supporting the body.

I failed to get photos for this exercise in time but wanted to include it, I do have a video available: go.cavemantraining.com/kbe-vid-132

# Kettlebell Folding Windmill

In this variation of the windmill, I took one part from the kettlebell armbar and combined it with a folding pattern, which is great for the hips. You can perform this while remaining kneeled and then fold, or you can come into hip extension and then fold, the latter provides more benefits for the hips. I will describe later.

How to perform:
1. Kneeling position
2. Lean forward
3. Curl the weight into the rack using both arms
4. Sit back into kneeling position
5. Press the weight overhead
6. Extend the hips
7. Sit back and perform a similar movement to what you would in a standing windmill
8. Bring the hand to the ground
9. Bend the elbow as you lower further and sit back
10. Create thoracic rotation
11. Keep your sight on the kettlebell
12. Come as low to the ground as possible
13. Pull yourself back up with the hip extensors
14. Press the hand into the ground
15. Come into full hip extension
16. Either lower to the knees or perform another repetition


I failed to get photos for this exercise in time but wanted to include it, I do have a video available: go.cavemantraining.com/kbe-vid-132

# Additional Information

The following sections are additional supporting information for kettlebell training.

## Mind-muscle Connection

Movement just happens, you will it and it's done. This is true in a way, some are lucky to have correctly performed a movement so many times it just comes naturally. But throw in a new movement or change an existing movement up and it's a different story.

Mind muscle connection is extremely important, it allows you to recruit more muscles for a movement, the right muscles, and it allows you to isolate muscles for a movement, i.e. purposely not recruit those muscles that <u>can</u> power the movement. It allows you to focus on the muscles you want to work harder and isolate. A great example I'll always go back to is the overhand wide grip pull-up. This exercise can be executed through contraction of many muscles with the main ones being the latissimus dorsi and elbow flexors. Creating elbow flexion when hanging from a bar would bring the shoulders to the bar as the angle in the elbow joints decrease and the hands are not moving away from the bar. Contraction of the lats pulls the elbows toward the hips, i.e. shoulder adduction which in turn will also pull the shoulders to the bar. I repeat again, there are many more muscles involved, like pectoralis major, teres major/minor, infraspinatus, even the triceps brachii long head, etc. but for this example, let's focus on the elbow flexors and lats. Here's where the magic of MMC helps, connect with your elbow flexors and relax them, connect with your lats and contract them, perform the movement with an isolation of the lats and you're truly working on strengthening the lats.

Another example, also with the pull-up. I see many of my athletes start out with not being able to connect with the lats to do a pull-up, they're mainly using the elbow flexors for the pull-up and if not fixed they can quickly develop tendinitis in the elbow flexors. To get them to connect with their lats I will tap the areas which they need to activate and I'll also perform a drill in which the visuals clearly demonstrate whether they're using the lats or elbow flexors.

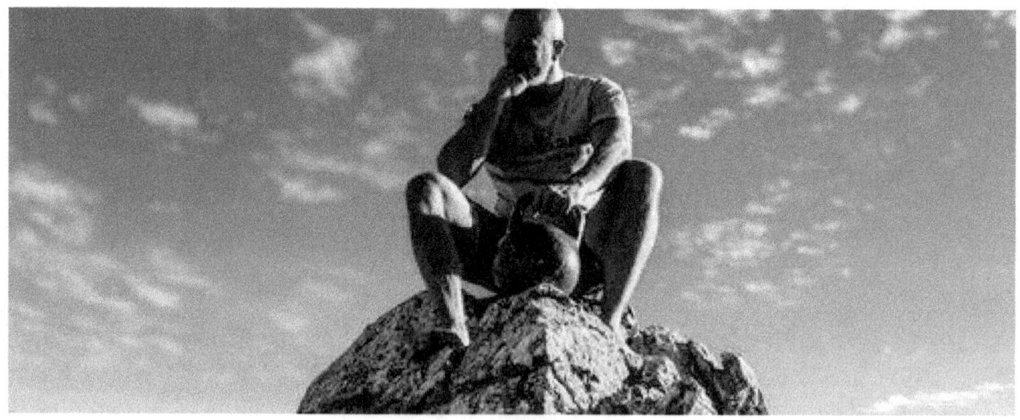

"If an exercise is done with good form, the right muscles do their job automatically." Incorrect. Are the right muscles really doing their work? Are we perhaps talking about an exercise which was progressed to properly with MMC involving all the muscles required, and was that exercise then repeated for high reps over a long period of time? Was that movement and contraction then stored only to be easily recalled and actioned without much thought?  I've also been told "but if I squat right now I just do it without much thought", ok, you might be flopping into what you believe is a good squat, or you've done it so many times that yes, you're working with something that has become second nature to do, but… Let's connect with your toes, the balls of your feet, external hip rotation, each of the three gluteals, hip flexors and extensors for pure alignment throughout, let's connect with the muscles around the scapulae for good spinal alignment, and so on. In fact, you do it right now, perform a fast squat as you're used to doing, then **slow down** and pick one of those areas I mentioned and include them through connection. At first you'll need to focus and connect, over time and when performed in high reps the body will get accustomed to it. Progression is again the key here. Slow and with thought. Practice, drill, and repeat, which over time will stick and allow you to go faster with more load.


A great example of connection loss is the toes, with a lot of people it's impossible for them to move their toes separately or at all. This is because the majority of shoes take away the ability to use them through soles that don't easily bend or shoe widths that cramp the toes together which take away the ability to use them for support or balance. Over many years the mind simply does not think about them anymore other than them being ten pieces of flesh hanging from our feet that are nice to decorate with colors. Free them, connect with them, train them, progress them, and over time it becomes natural.

## Kettlebell Anatomy

1.  Handle
2.  Corner(s)
3.  Horn(s)
4.  Window
5.  Bell AKA body
6.  Base

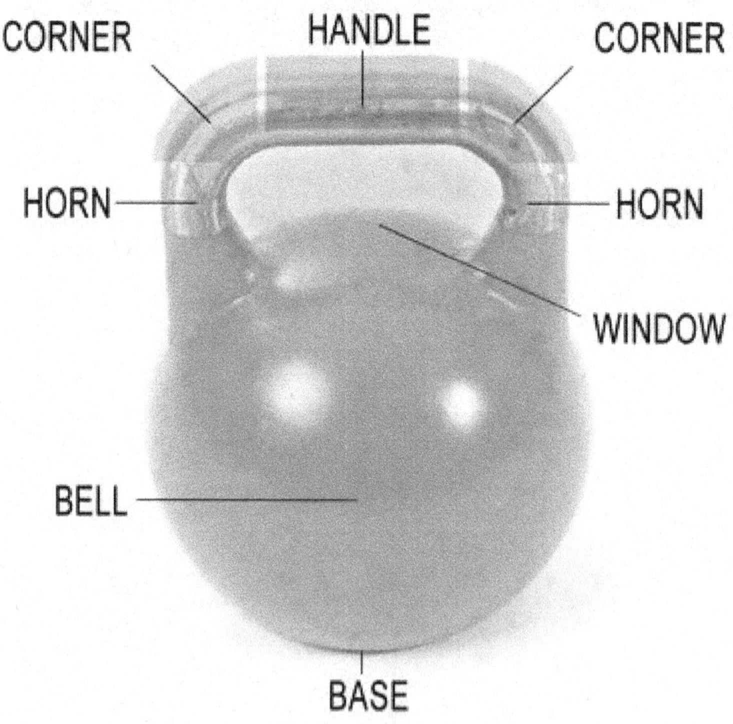

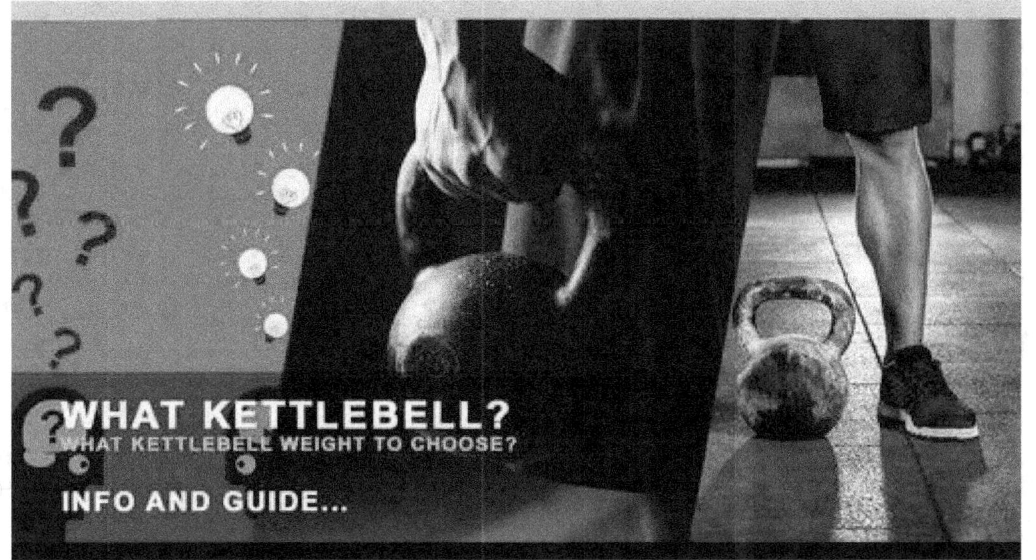


## What Weight Kettlebell Should I Start With?

Let's say you're limited to buying one kettlebell, you want to make sure you buy the right kettlebell. **How do you decide what kettlebell weight to choose?**

Kettlebells are not cheap, so you want to make sure you buy the right weight, which will allow you to get the most out of your one kettlebell. Here are some tips to start thinking about what kettlebell weight to choose.

### Goals?

What are your goals, why are you buying a kettlebell?

- Lose weight/fat loss
- Gain overall strength
- Become flexible
- Increase cardiovascular endurance
- Etc.

Based on those answers you can compile the exercises you'll mainly want to be doing. Performing a racked squat with a kettlebell is completely different from a ballistic swing, or overhead reverse lunge.

Are you going to be performing high reps, or low reps, swinging 20, 50, 100 or more, or in sets of 6 to 12? If you can handle a 24kg swing, that doesn't mean it's the right weight to use for high volume or endurance. You'll want to go at least 1/3 lower to what your submax is.

If you're mainly going to be doing slow lifts and carries like, deadlifts, farmer walks, racked walks, goblet squats, racked squats, and even some double-arm chest presses etc. you can go considerably higher with the weight. Let's say you would get a 16kg if you were going to swing a lot, then you could easily get a 24 to 28kg for these types of exercises.

If you want to work on endurance or cardio, you'll be doing a higher volume, if you want to work on strength, hypertrophy, then you'll be doing lower volume.

## Current State?

What is your current state, how strong, flexible, fit are you? If you've never touched a weight in your life before, then you'll need a different weight than someone who has been going to the gym for years.

**Are you very inflexible?** If so, this will also affect the weight you choose. You'll run more risk of injury if you're inflexible, hence you'll need to reduce the weight and focus on flexibility more.

## Experience?

Have you already got some experience with lifting barbells, dumbbells, etc.? If so, it will be easier to understand some of the concepts in kettlebell training, hence, you'll be safer, so you can increase the weight you choose. But, you should still take into consideration that the kettlebell has a different weight distribution than the barbell or dumbbell, this will make the kettlebell feel much heavier, i.e. if you're pressing a 30kg dumbbell 1RM, you'll need to subtract 4kg or more for a kettlebell, as you won't be able to transfer the exact amount to a kettlebell.

Have you got no experience what so ever with a kettlebell or any other weight? You should seriously consideration this, and start at the low end. Safety first.

## Guide

Following is a guide on what kettlebell weight to choose, however, you should consider all the points above first and make your own informed decision.

| Lots of overhead work | Male | | Female | |
|---|---|---|---|---|
| | Low Volume | High Volume | Low Volume | High Volume |
| Never done anything overhead | 8 to 12kg | 8 to 10kg | 8kg | 8kg |
| Mediocre with overhead work | 12 to 16kg | 12kg | 12kg | 10kg |
| Do overhead work in the gym regularly | 16 to 20kg | 16kg | 16kg | 12kg |

| Lots of slow lifts | Male | | Female | |
|---|---|---|---|---|
| | Low Volume | High Volume | Low Volume | High Volume |
| Never done any slow lifts | 16kg | 12kg | 12kg | 10kg |
| Mediocre with slow lifts | 20 to 24kg | 16kg | 18kg | 16kg |
| Do slow lifts in the gym regularly | 24 to 32kg | 20kg | 24kg | 20kg |

| Lots of ballistic work | Male | | Female | |
|---|---|---|---|---|
| | Low Volume | High Volume | Low Volume | High Volume |
| Never done anything ballistic | 12 to 16kg | 12kg | 12kg | 10kg |
| Mediocre with ballistic work | 16 to 20kg | 16kg | 16kg | 14kg |
| Do ballistic work in the gym regularly | 20 to 24kg | 20kg | 20kg | 16kg |

Still not sure? Buy an online assessment, discuss your goals, submit your video, get feedback, and a recommendation.

## Which Kettlebell to Choose and Why?

I'm a great advocate for competition kettlebells, even when not used for Kettlebell Sport. That said, I'll provide as much information about the different kettlebells available, so you can make your own decision.

If you're just starting with kettlebell training, you'll want to start with something light, so that you can focus on form and technique. Starting with a weight that is too heavy will compromise your form and technique, and potentially cause injury.

Differences:

- Handle diameter
- Handle shape
- Window diameter
- Base diameter
- Bell dimension
- Weight
- Colour
- Coat
  - Neoprene
  - Rubber
  - Vinyl
  - Powder
- Material
  - Steel
  - Iron
- Filling
  - Sand
  - Water
  - Hollow

Competition Kettlebells AKA Pro Grade Kettlebells, Sport Kettlebells, Girya Sport Kettlebell

Classic Kettlebells AKA Iron-cast Kettlebells

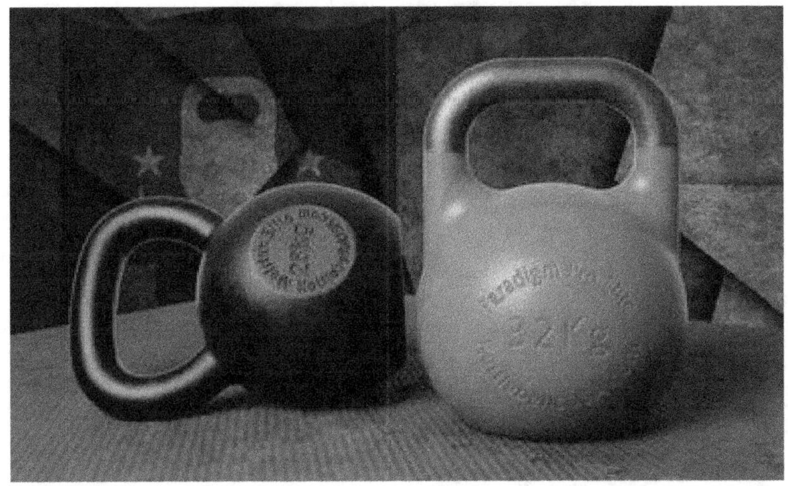

*Cast-iron versus Steel Competition Kettlebell*

**Classic Kettlebells are less expensive than the Competition Kettlebells.**

As mentioned earlier, my preference is the Competition Kettlebell and the reason for that is the competition kettlebell remains the same size, no matter what weight you work with; whether it's an 8kg or 24kg, the size of the kettlebell remains the same. This is a great feature because there is no need to get used to different shapes and sizes when you go up in weight. Furthermore, the base of the comp kettlebell is a lot wider, allowing you to do things like burpee deadlifts, renegade rows, and other exercises where you need to place your weight on the kettlebell - a narrow base has the potential for the bell to topple over and cause wrist injury. I find it difficult to find comfortable positions with the classic kettlebells, especially the lighter weight.

Rubber, neoprene, and vinyl-coated kettlebells are more suitable for surfaces that scratch or chip easily. Vinyl is harder and more resistant to damage than rubber. Neoprene is softer than both rubber and vinyl, which increases comfort. All that said, I've not had good experience with these type of coated kettlebells myself.

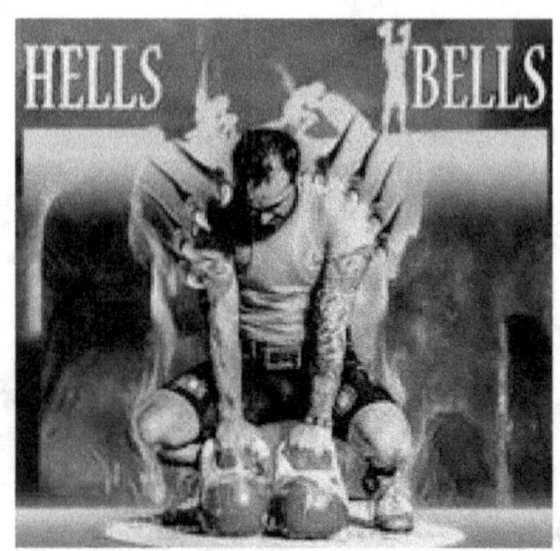

*David Keohan*

International Kettlebell Colour Standard for Competition Kettlebells:

| Weight in Kilos | Weight in Pounds | Colour |
| --- | --- | --- |
| 8 | 17.6 (order) | Pink |
| 12 | 26.4 (order) | Blue |
| 16 | 35.2 (order) | Yellow |
| 20 | 44.0 (order) | Purple |
| 24 | 52.8 (order) | Green |
| 28 | 61.6 (order) | Orange |
| 32 | 70.4 (order) | Red |
| 36 | 79.2 (order) | Grey |
| 40 | 88.0 (order) | White |
| 44 | 96.8 (order) | Silver |
| 48 | 105.6 | Gold |

There are also weights in between (for example, 10 kg, 14 kg, and so on), and these are usually colored with a different shade of the neighboring weight, or defined by a black band on the handle.

## What Weight to Choose?

The weight you choose for training depends on your goals and what exercises you will primarily be doing with it, in addition to your current strength. If we're talking primarily about double-arm swings done by absolute beginners, I'd suggest 8kg or less for children, 10kg to 12kg for adolescents, 12kg for women, and 14 to 16kg for men.

For overhead pressing, I suggest at least 4 to 6kg less than mentioned for the swings above. For chest pressing, 2 to 4kg less, as most people are stronger with chest presses compared to overhead presses.

For rowing with the focus being on the rear deltoids, I suggest the same weight as for swings or even slightly more weight. For rows that focus more on the middle of the back, I suggest the same weight as for overhead presses.

For deadlifts, squat style, I suggest the same as swings or more, and possibly even double kettlebells. For deadlifts hip hinge, I recommend the same as swings or slightly less.

That covers the basic exercises. If you're talking about any other exercise, you've already progressed and are more than likely able to make an informed decision on what weight to use.

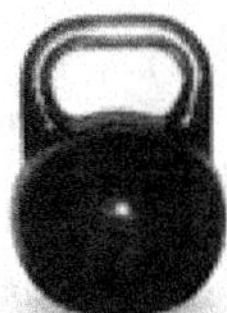 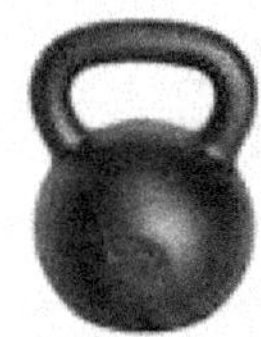 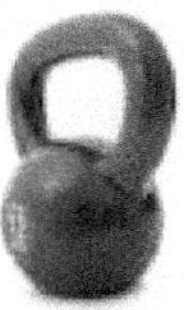 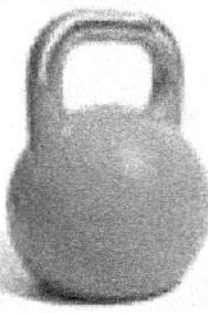

## Where to Buy Kettlebells Online

Out of the many places to buy kettlebells online, you'll see the following names and brands pop up the most: Amazon, Kettlebell Kings, DragonDoor/RKC, Onnit, Agatsu, Ader, Kettlebells USA.

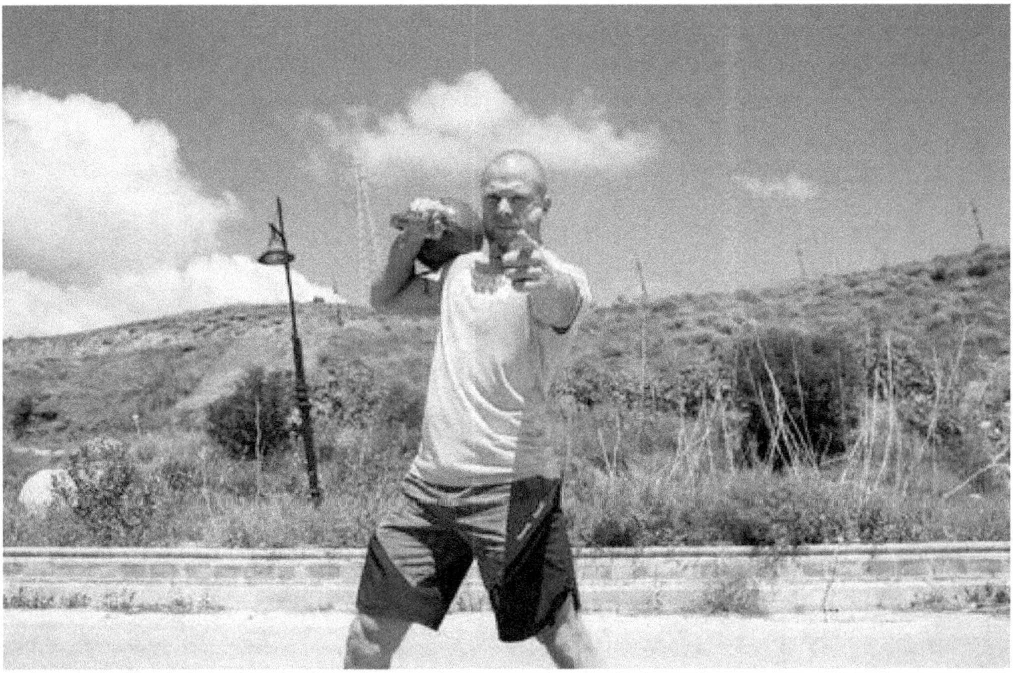

# Kettlebell Grips

There are many different types of kettlebell grips you will need to employ during kettlebell training, the following are photos and basic explanations of what each different grip is used for. If you enrolled in one of our <u>free or paid online kettlebell courses</u> you will see these different grips referred to.

**Important:** with each grip, there are only one or two exercises listed to get a general idea across, but in most cases, there are many more than those listed.  Grips might differ slightly across kettlebells, as the width of the handle increases with some of the classic kettlebells when the weight goes up.

Along your kettlebell journey, you will find that different associations or organizations will use different grips for different exercises, and as long as it works and is safe, there is nothing wrong with it.

For illustration purposes, a competition kettlebell is used, which changes in weight but not in size.

Note that these are **not** barbell grips, as the names might be the same, the technique is not.

*"excellent document and the content is highly accurate"*
*~ Valerie Pawlowski World Champion Kettlebell Lifting*

**General Information**

The following rules and tips apply in general to most kettlebell grips. A grip on the kettlebell handle or horns should almost never be tight, it should be as loose as possible without losing grip of the kettlebell and conserving as much grip strength without burning out the muscles.

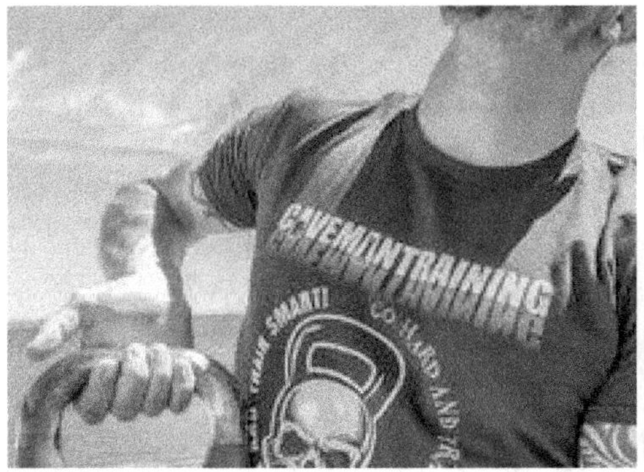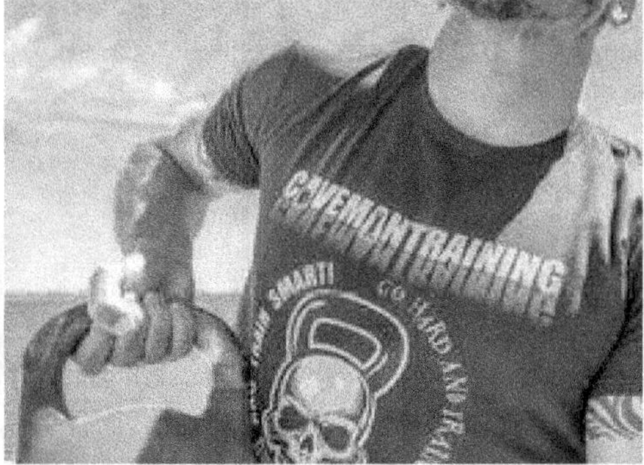

*Loose versus tight grip*

**Blisters** usually occur when the skin is folded within the grip, especially when using heavy weights or doing high volume reps. Try and slide your fingers around the handle or horns while keeping skin folds from occurring and then close the grip. Another cause for blisters is friction, avoid friction by proper kettlebell guidance (which you'll learn in our courses).

**Ripped calluses** usually occur when there is friction within the palms, biggest culprit is kettlebell bobbing, to prevent the kettlebell from bobbing search for my article online 'kettlebell swing insert', the insert prevents the kettlebell from doing a full pendulum which is usually causing abrupt stopping of the kettlebell.

*"You should look at it like this. If you're making the pendulum movement and let the bell go where it wants to go, it abruptly gets stopped by your body, i.e. your arms hit your thighs or whatever part of the body, the bell will want to keep going, this is creating the friction in your hands, on high reps or heavyweight this will cause blisters.*

*To fix, think about directing the weight to the back, create a deep insert, think first part of the swing PENDULUM and then bang, INSERT. Direct the weight to the back. Hope that helps."*

The most **common grip** and **transition** are that from hook grip to loose grip which occurs during the clean and rack, the hook grip is also used for single-arm swings and snatches, the second most common grip is the double hand grip which is used for double arm swings.

This transition is one that beginners should focus on, the need to want to hold the kettlebell handle tight, and perform no transition is high with beginners. This is such an important concept that everyone should spend a lot of time on until they get it right. I can highly recommend performing assisted cleans to work on this.

## Why should you learn about grips?

It is important to know and understand kettlebell grips for efficiency and being able to work the muscles intended for the exercise in question. Employing an incorrect grip can mean pain; being uncomfortable; cause for injury; exhausting grip, forearm, biceps or shoulder muscles and losing focus on the muscles targeted with a specific exercise.

## Why use different grips?

If you're asking this question, then you're asking the right question because knowing a lot of grips is cool, but knowing why you would change grip or use one over the other is even  cooler and the part you should really understand.

During kettlebell training, you employ different grips to make certain exercises more efficient, but you also change grips to increase difficulty and challenge other muscle groups. Sometimes when your training gets stale you might even employ a different grip to please the mind.

While knowing kettlebell grips and when to employ them is important and one of the kettlebell fundamentals, the second most important thing you should start looking into is racking a kettlebell. It might seem insignificant, but a lot hinges on how you rack your kettlebell, in fact, some people give up on kettlebell training because they can't get comfortable in the racking position or can't find the proper position for the bell to rest.

Search Google for 'Cavemantraining Kettlebell Racking' to start learning about this next topic in kettlebell fundamentals.

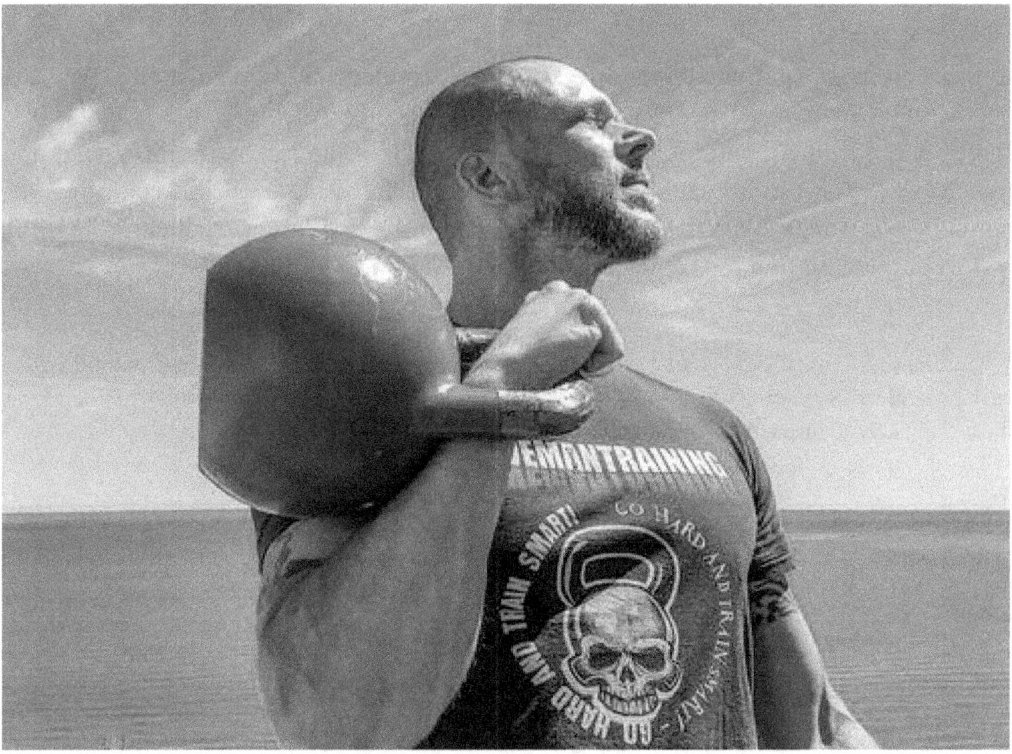

I invite you to watch a video on our YouTube channel which demonstrates several  kettlebell clean transitions into different grips go.cavemantraining.com/mkg-vid-1

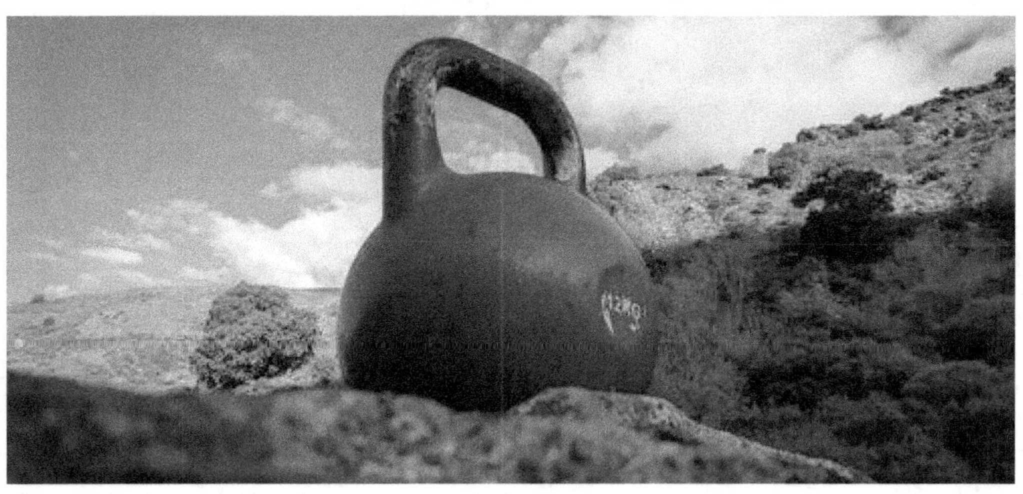

## 45-Degree Angle

In grips employed for **racking** or **pressing**, the handle should be positioned at a 45-degree angle within the palm, one corner positioned between the thumb and index finger, and the other corner is past the heel of the palm. The reason for this position is to keep the wrist straight and hand in line with the forearm, this will avoid pressure on the wrist. A bent wrist means there is a kink in the line through which power will be lost during pressing plus the cause for potential injury.

When working with a light kettlebell this might not be so noticeable, but when working with heavier kettlebells the pressure can be enormous, cause damage to the wrist and/or prevent you from being able to press the kettlebell up.

When people first start training with a kettlebell, you'll find that they employ the broken wrist grip to relieve the pressure that the bell provides on the forearm, this is especially so for new people who are not used to this pressure. You should take the person aside and have them play with the grip, handle position and bell positioning until they feel ok with the pressure of the kettlebell being in the correct position. You should also explain that it's quite normal to experience some mild discomfort until the area is more conditioned.

See illustrations below for correct 45-degree handle angle in the palm.

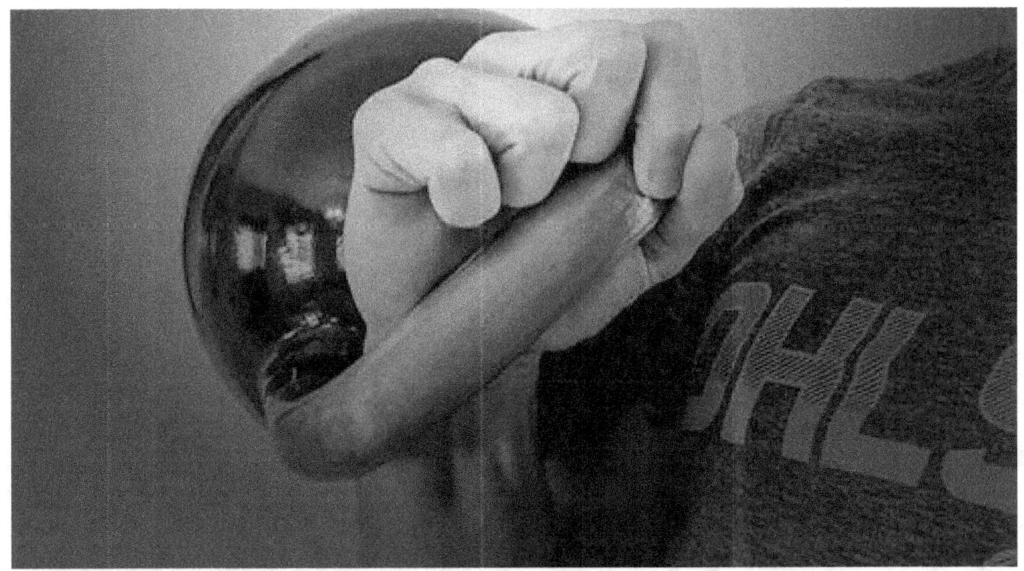

*Correct 45° angle of the handle within the palm*

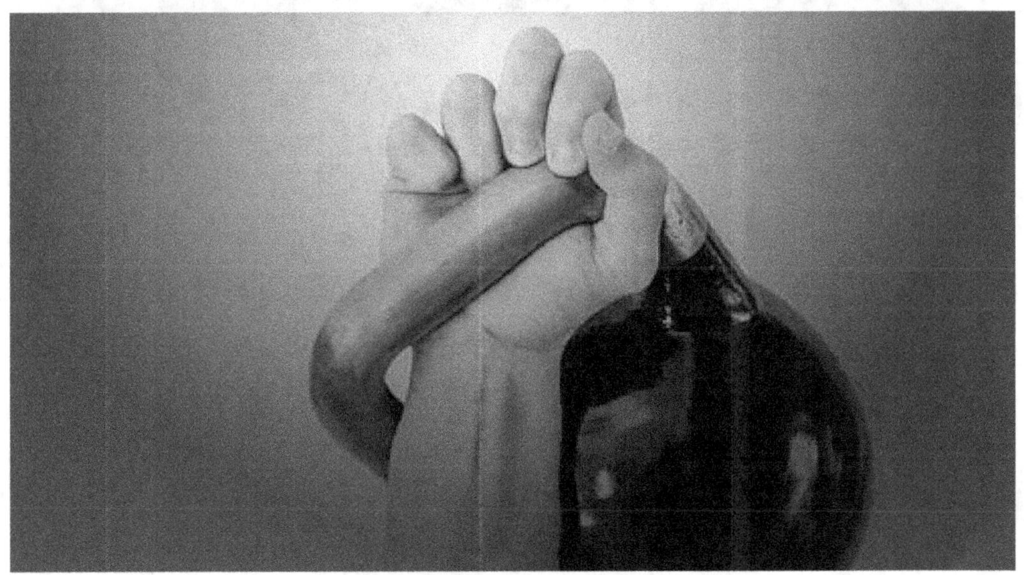

*Correct 45° angle of the handle within the palm*

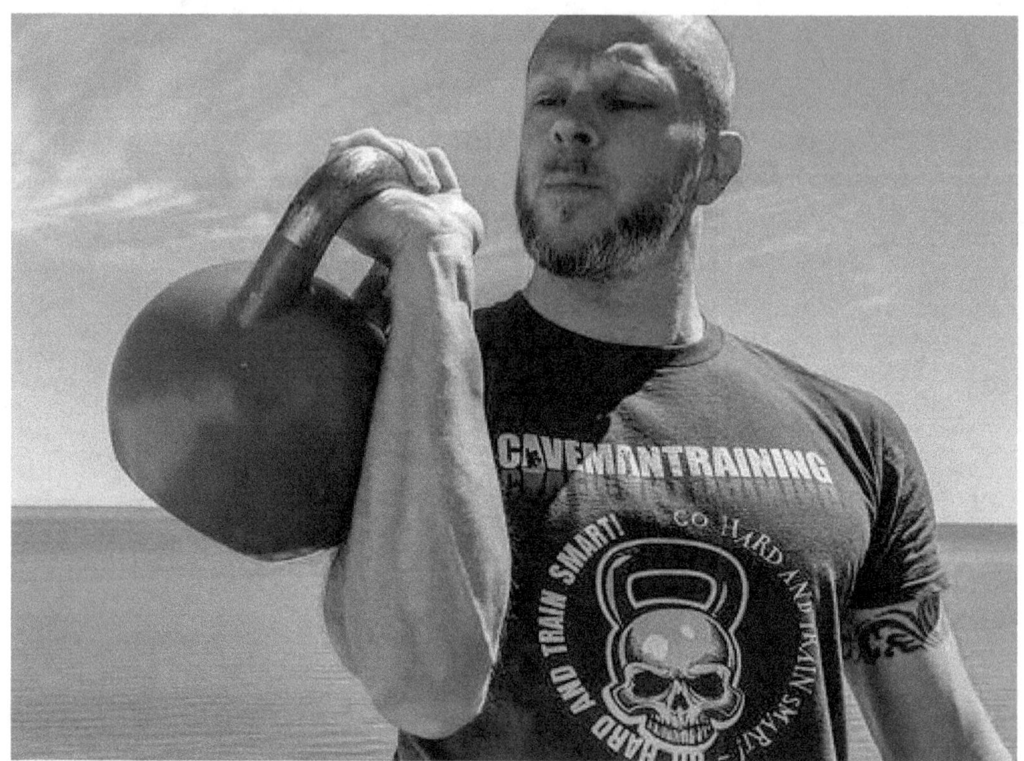

*Handle incorrectly positioned within the palm, AKA "broken wrist"
note that the left corner is not over the heel of the palm*

## Grip Categories

Grips can be categorized in the following categories:

- Pressing grips
- Racking grips
- Lifting grips
- Ballistic grips
- Juggling grips

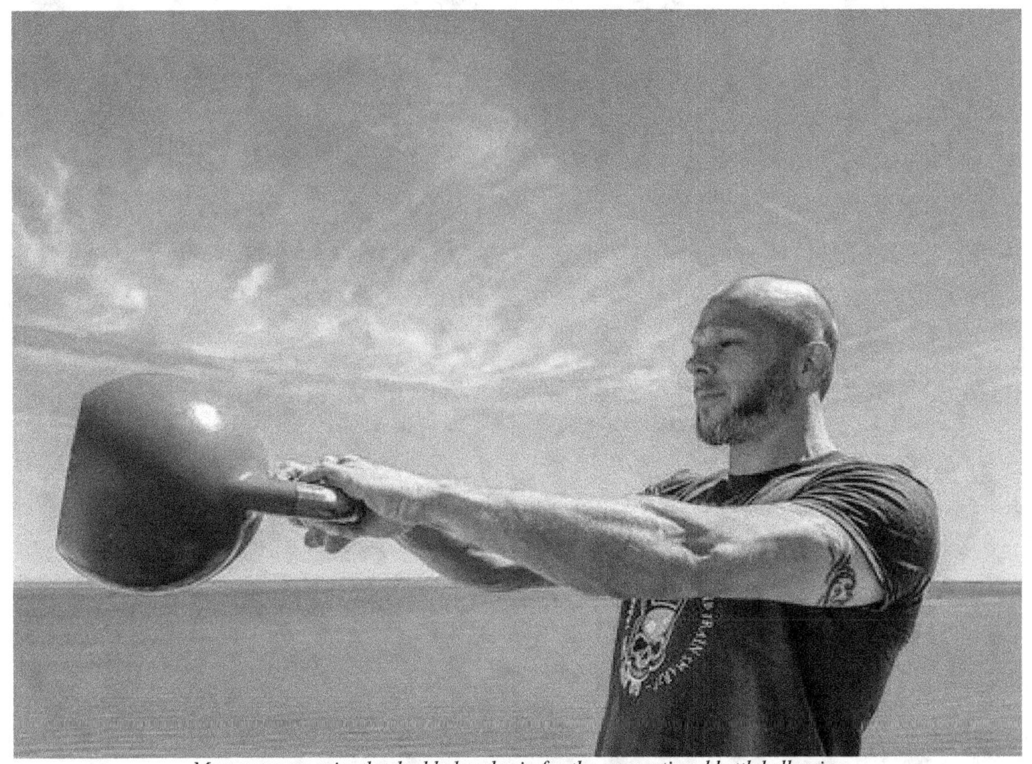

*Most common grip, the double hand grip for the conventional kettlebell swing*

## Broken Wrist Grip—incorrect grip

As the name implies, this is not a grip you'll want to employ. It's named so because the straight-line your arm and palm should be in is broken. A correct kettlebell grip is one of the main things to focus on when you start kettlebell training. You have to get it right, take some time away from everyone and take a light kettlebell, play with it, move it around till you find the two or three points in racking where the weight should rest. The resting points are; around the heel of the palm; on the forearm; and against the biceps when in cradle racking position.

When your wrist is not straight/neutral in racking or overhead position, all the weight is pulling down on your wrist. Most people employ this incorrect grip because they might feel less pressure on the forearm, however, one should take the time to find the right resting points to maintain a neutral wrist. The second cause for an incorrect grip/insert is a tight grip and not opening up during the clean for a proper hand insert.

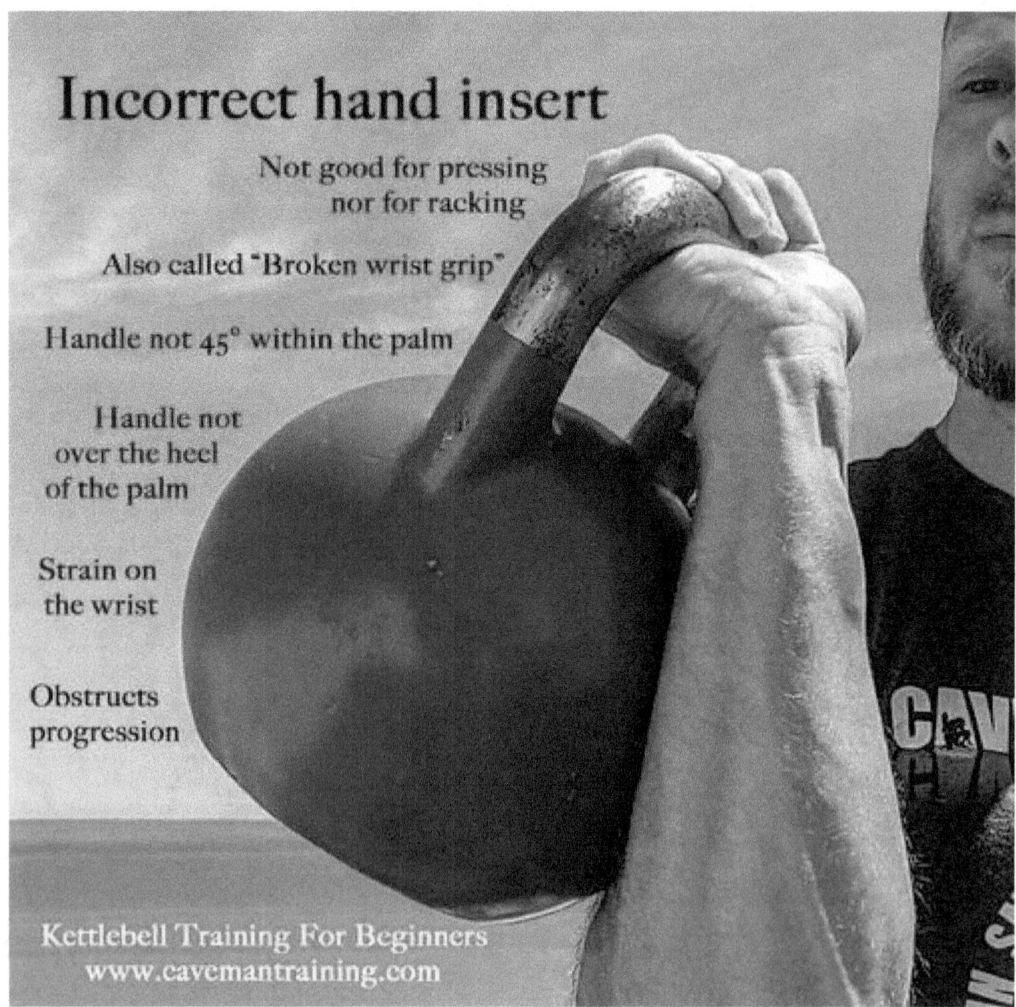

The above photo can be saved/shared on Facebook from the following link:

go.cavemantraining.com/mkg-link-1


The photo below can be saved/shared on Facebook from:

go.cavemantraining.com/mkg-link-2

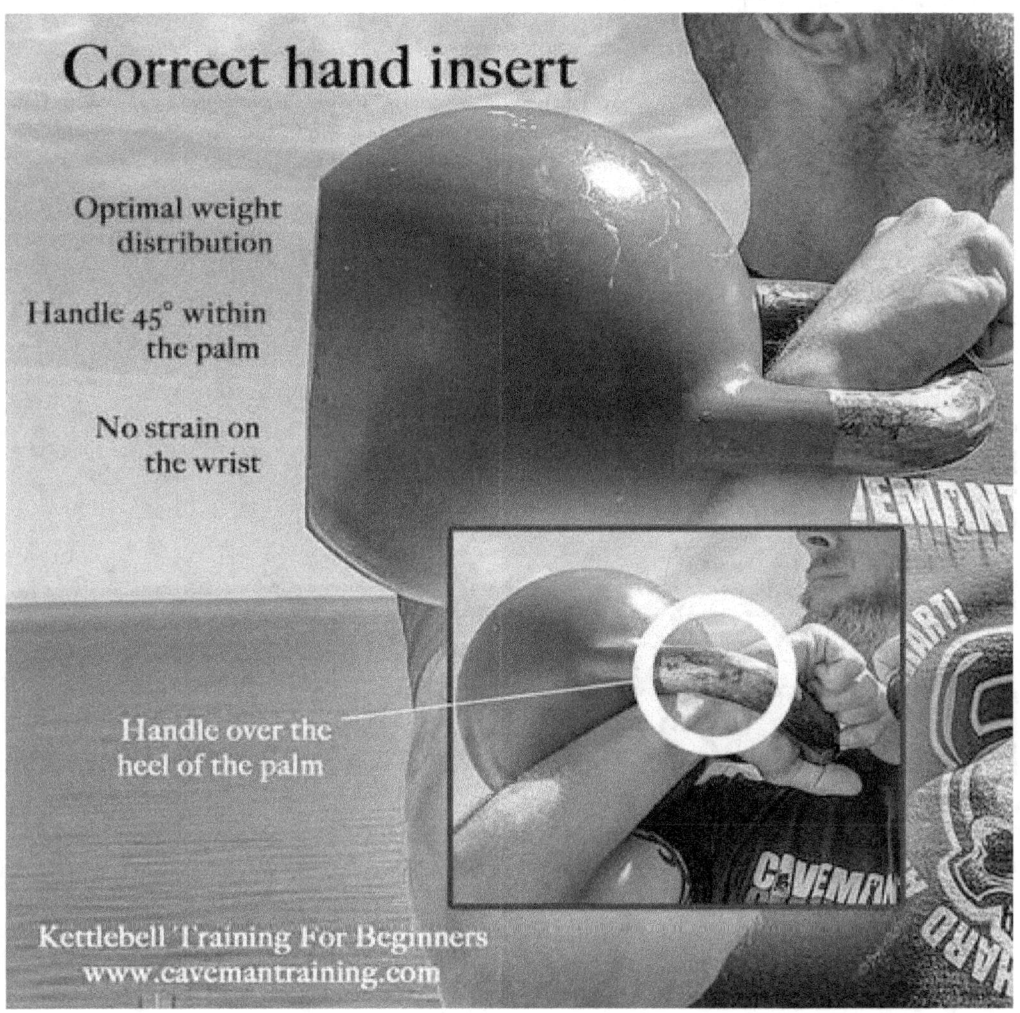

# Without further ado, let's dive deep into the kettlebell grips.

### Double Hand Grip

**Grip:** two hands, four fingers closed around the handle placed on the corners or horns depending on hand size and thumbs loose.

**Ideal for:** double-arm swings and deadlifts

This grip is mostly used for doing double arm swings and deadlifts. Like with most grips, do not turn this into a tight grip, keep some space for the handle to move freely without causing friction. This grip should loosen up at the top part of the swing to stop the grip from burning out. You will have eight fingers around the handle, with big hands your fingers might feel squashed when doing high volume reps, pay particular attention to the ring fingers at high volume reps as they'll be prone to blisters.

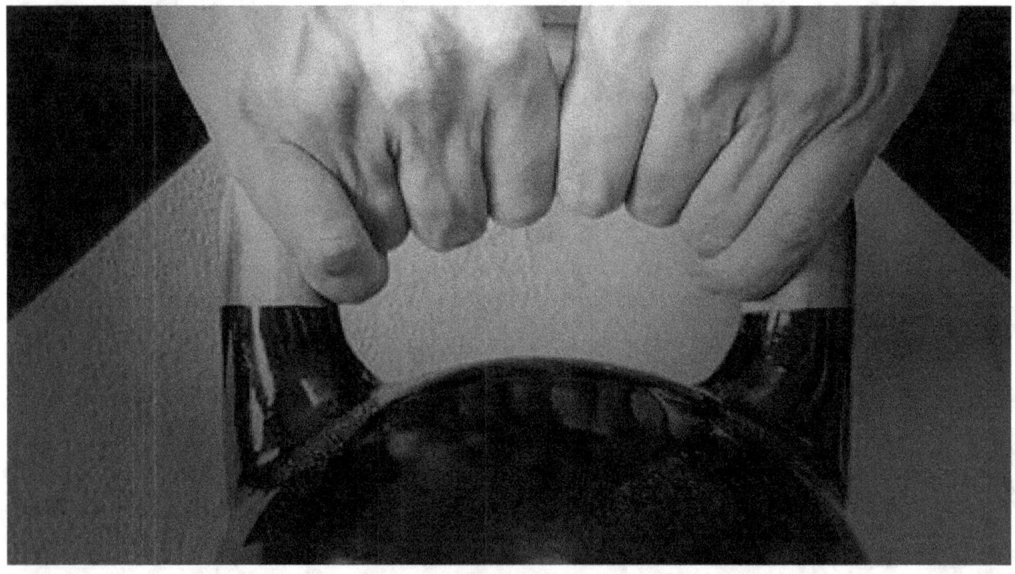

The grip can be employed with both of the pinkies positioned within the horns *(pictured above)* or over the horns *(pictured further below under the Closed Double Hand Grip)*.

## Swan Grip

This grip is used primarily in rowing drills and pulling or front holding movements.

Grasping with fingers mostly straight in a beak like hold over top of kettlebell with arm bent at wrist and elbow in "S" like position, as that of swan neck, with emphasis on squeeze of fingers and strong forearm engagement this grip works tremendous grip strength for massive finger and forearm recruitment.

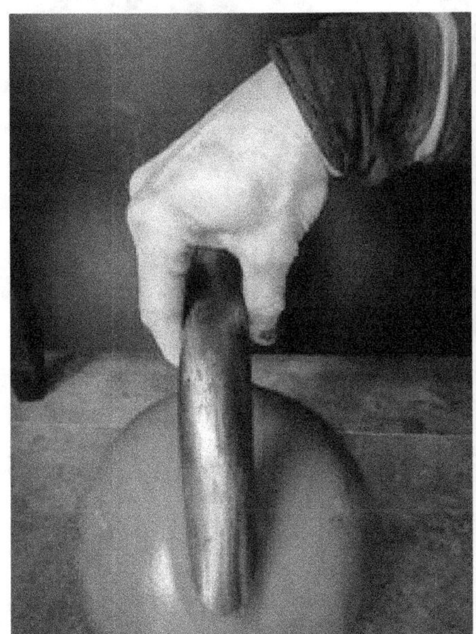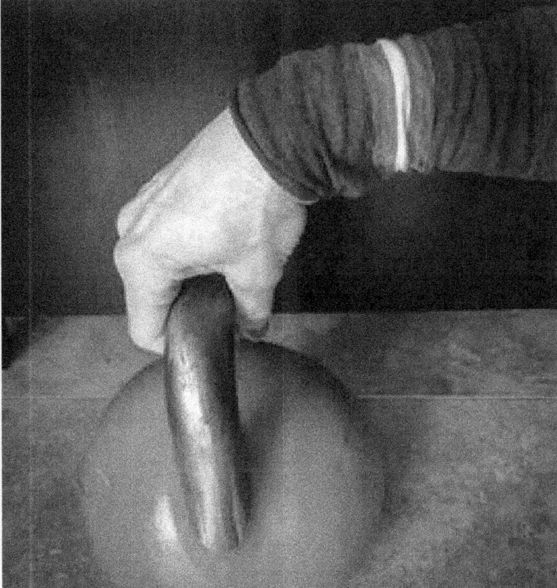

*Swan grip*

## OK Grip (AKA 2 or 3 Finger Grip)

With thumb and first finger (and middle for 3) in an 2 finger lock wrap around handle. Remaining 3 fingers are off or relaxed (2 off on the ok 3 hold) away from handle.

Useful for carries, swings, clean or row. The thumb and first finger are the most important to primary grip strength. Working with these variations puts attention on the longer lasting strength to hang on to the fullest extent especially digging out on final Snatches.

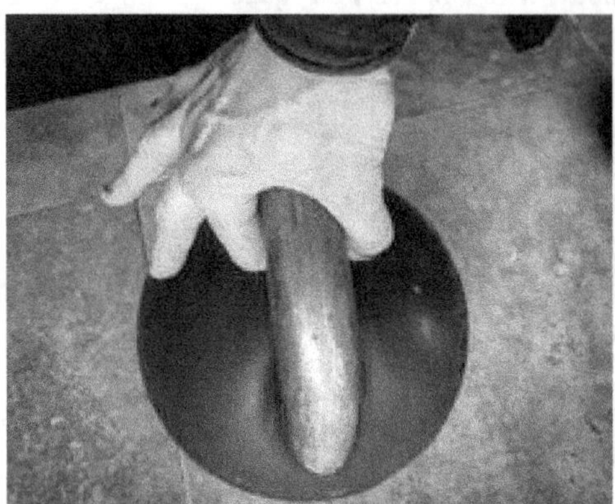 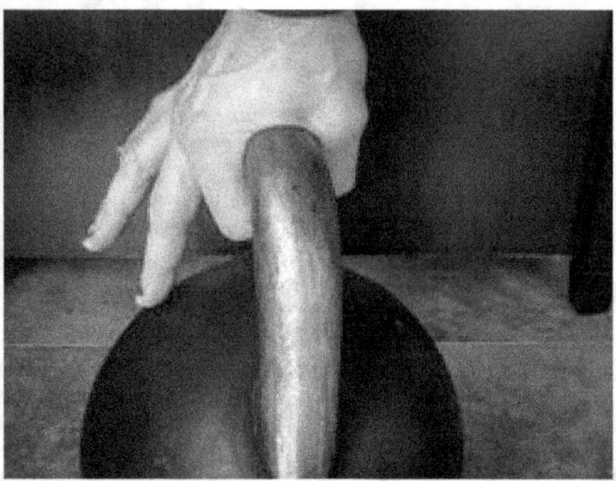

*Ok grip*
*Thanks to Valerie Pawlowski for the photos and information.*

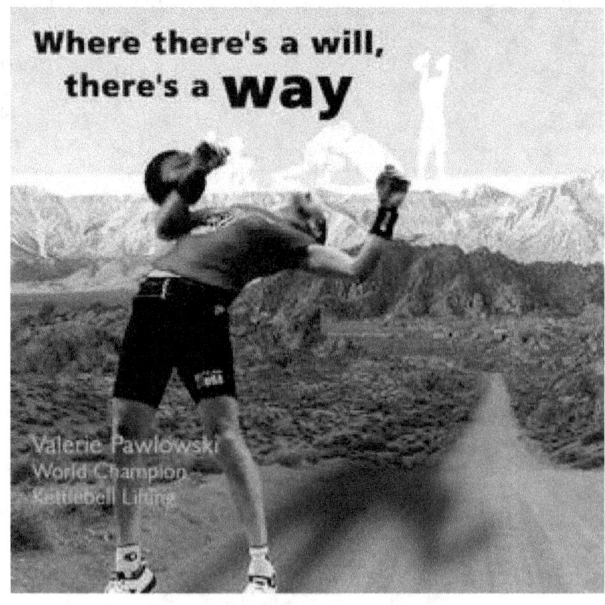

## Double Hand Corkscrew Grip

**Grip:** same as the double hand grip but with the horns between the pinkie and ring fingers.


**Ideal for:** double-arm swings and American swings

This is a grip I've started using when doing heavy high volume swings during the **Caveman Kettlebells 28 Day Swing Challenge**, which I like to call the Double Hand Corkscrew Grip because it's very similar to a grip on a corkscrew, when holding a corkscrew, the screw itself will be positioned between the middle finger and ring finger, but with the kettlebell the horn will be positioned between the ring finger and pinkie. Everything from the Double Hand Grip transfers to this grip. I like to use this grip to switch it up, but also because I have big hands and usually need to put my pinkies over the handles with the Double Hand Grip, with this grip I feel that my fingers are less squashed. It is very important to wrap your pinkies around the horn to prevent them from getting caught in your clothes during the swing. This grip also provides more stability at the top of the American swing and helps prevent skin tears on the outside of the pinkie.

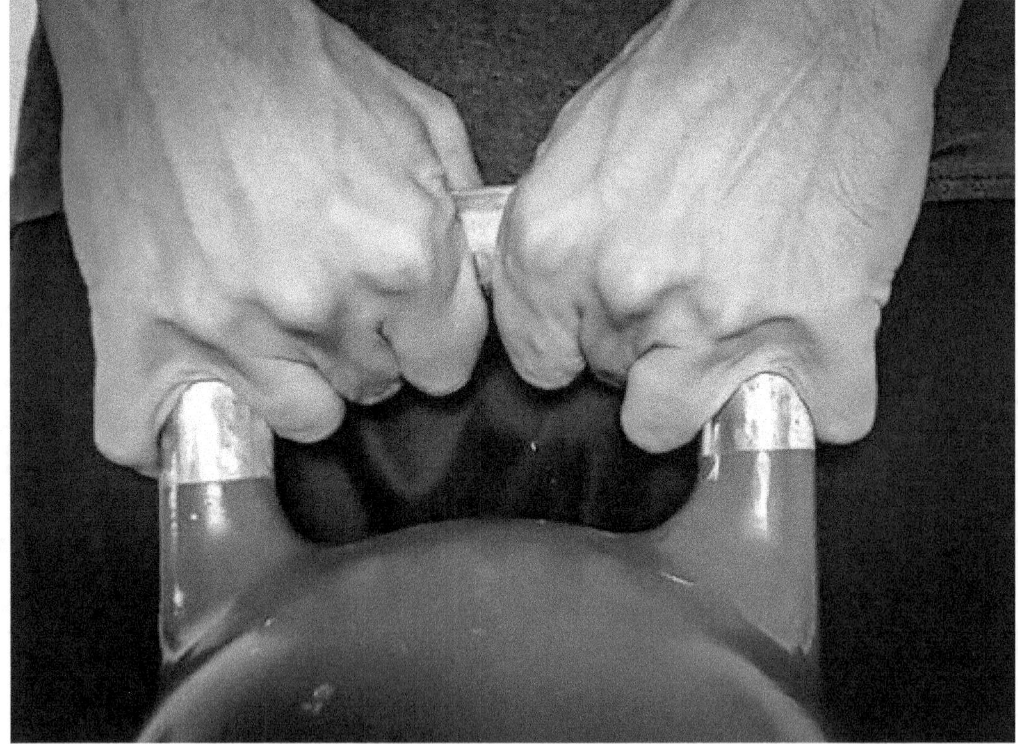

*Double hand corkscrew grip*

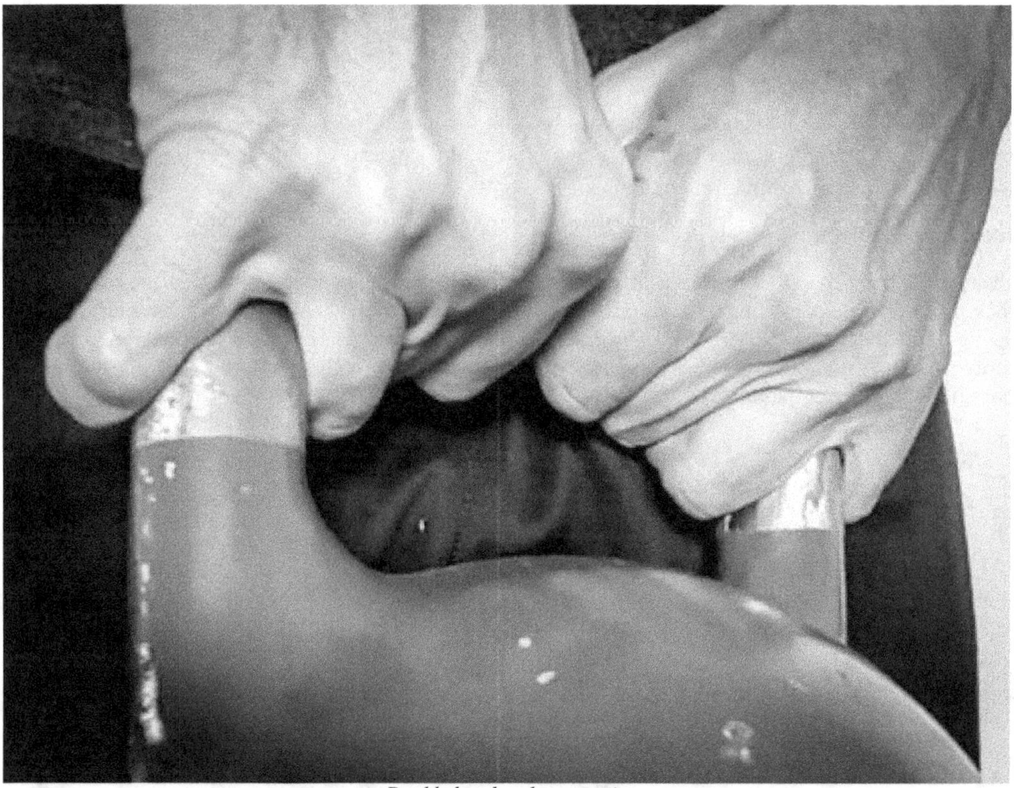

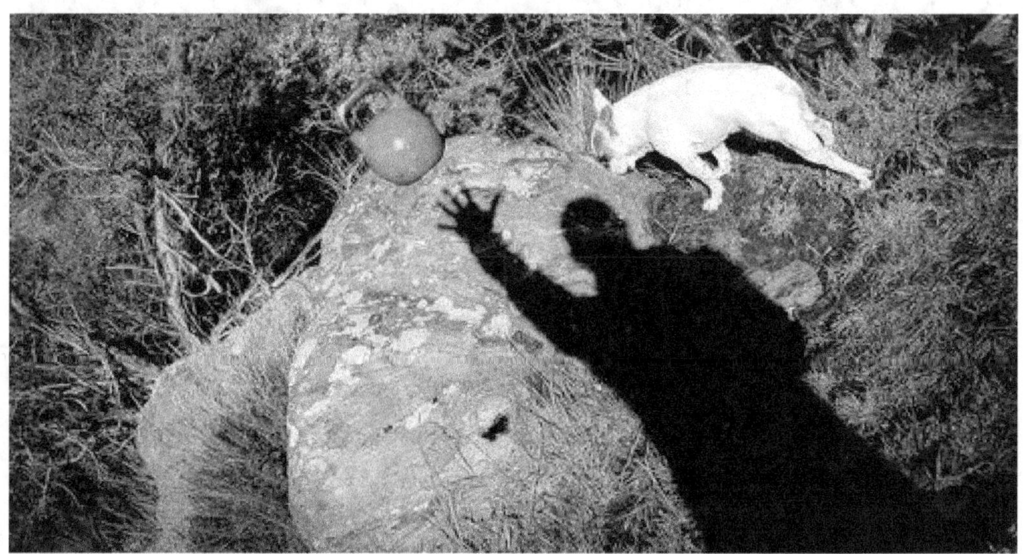

*Double hand corkscrew grip*

*Come and say "hi" in our 11,000+ strong Facebook group* www.facebook.com/groups/KettlebellTraining

## Closed Double Hand Grip

**Handle:** two hands, four fingers and thumbs locking the index finger down, or locking both the index and middle finger down. Can also be with the pinkies over the horns as illustrated below, in which case it becomes, three fingers plus lock.

**Ideal for:** double-arm swings, deadlifts

Everything from the Double Hand Grip transfers to this grip, the difference is that the thumbs are locking over the index fingers, this grip is for using extremely heavy weights, or high volume swings and the grip is giving up. The lock is also employed to relieve some tension from the forearms. The lock might also be possible with one thumb two fingers. Note: this grip might not be possible with thicker handles.

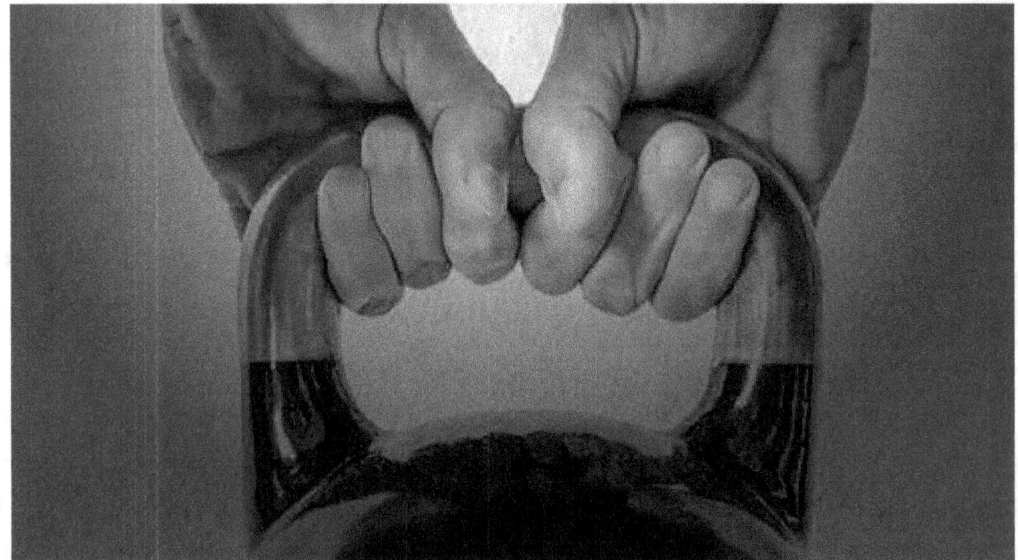

*Closed double hand grip*

## Hook Grip (AKA Overhand Grip)

**Handle:** one hand, four fingers and thumb loose

**Ideal for:** down-phase of most ballistic movements, dead clean

With this grip, the handle is positioned within the fingers which are bend, used when the Kettlebell travels downwards for single arm swings and downward phase of snatches. Note that the thumb can move over to the other side of the handle *(but not locking finger)* and the hand is positioned closer to one side of the handle.

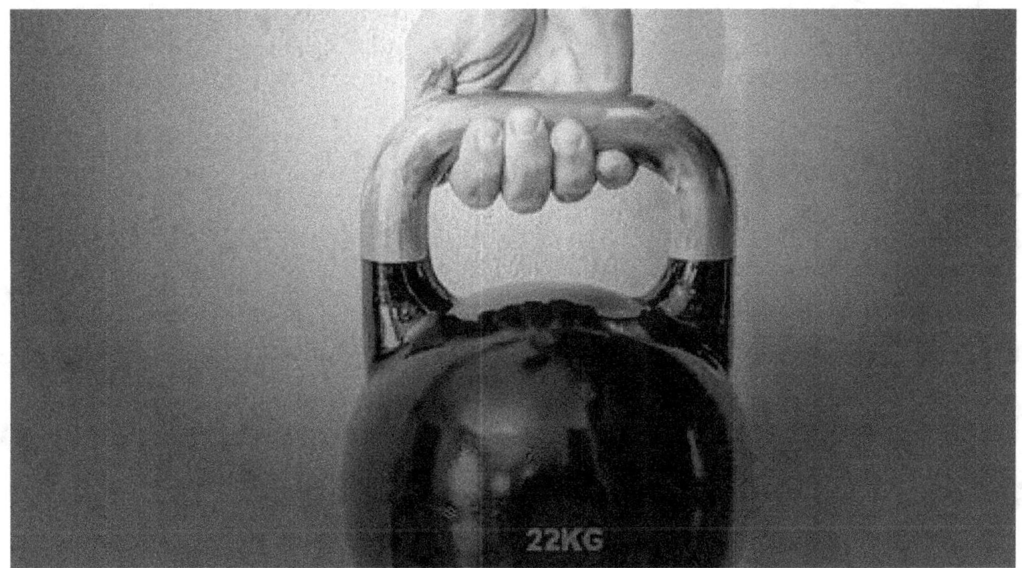

Closed Hook Grip (AKA C grip)

**Handle:** one hand, four fingers and thumb locking the index finger down, or both the index and middle finger

**Ideal for:** single-arm swings, snatch, dead clean

This grip is the same as the Hook Grip apart from there being a finger lock with the thumb over forefinger. The lock provides a better grip but also releases tension on the forearms and fingers. If you experience fingers cramps, forearms pains or soreness, try switching to a closed hook grip. Issues arise especially when just starting out with training or when doing high volume reps without implementing a closed grip.

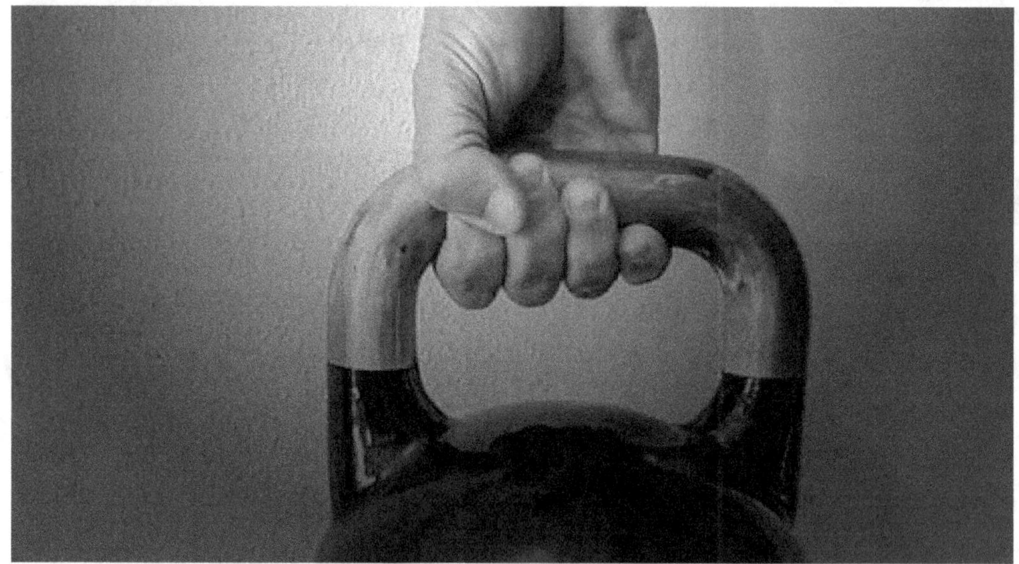

## Racking Grip

This is the common grip employed in racking position with a closed but relaxed fist, fingers gently resting on the handle. If you work with two kettlebells you should look at employing the racking safety grip.

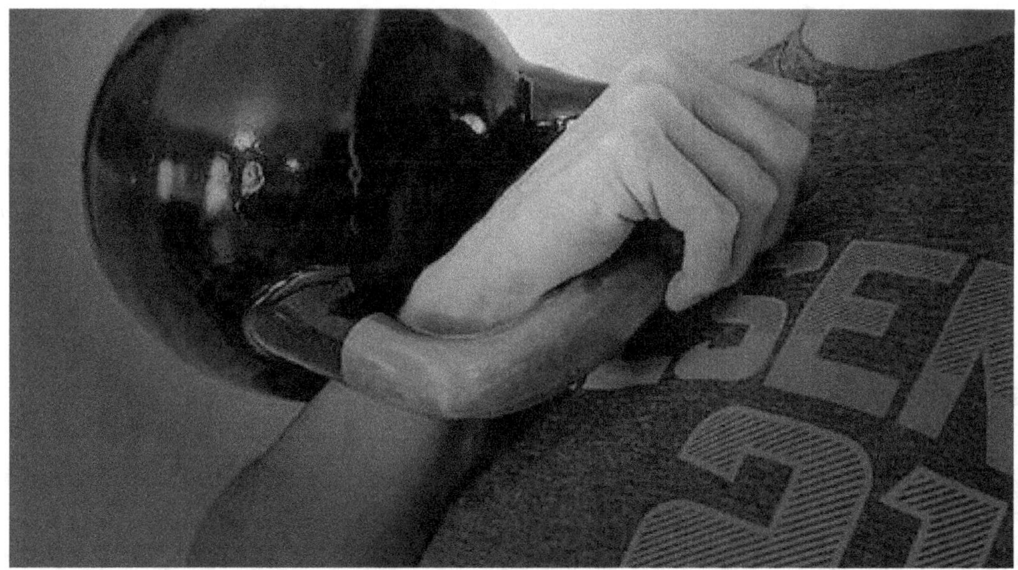

Racking is important for resting, pressing, squatting and all require a different type of rack. Search Google for 'Cavemantraining Kettlebell Racking' to get the free info on racking.

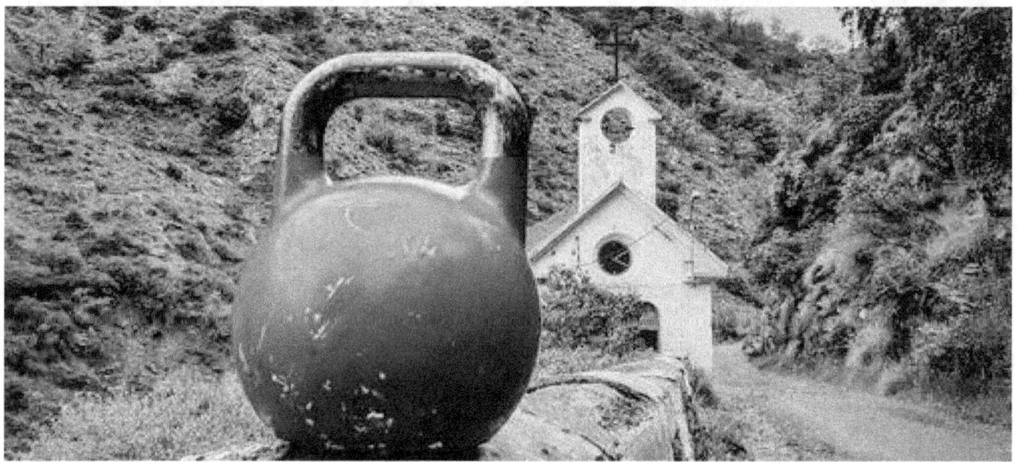

## Racking Safety Grip

With this grip the thumb is over the index finger which are placed over the horn, and the remaining fingers are tucked behind the handle, this grip is used when working with Two kettlebells to protect the fingers from getting caught between the two kettlebell handles.

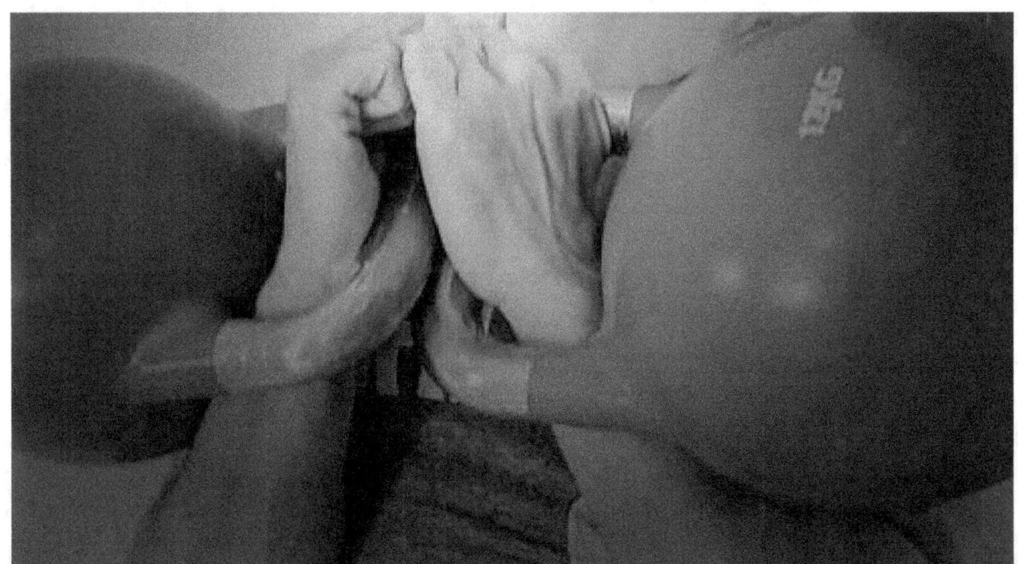

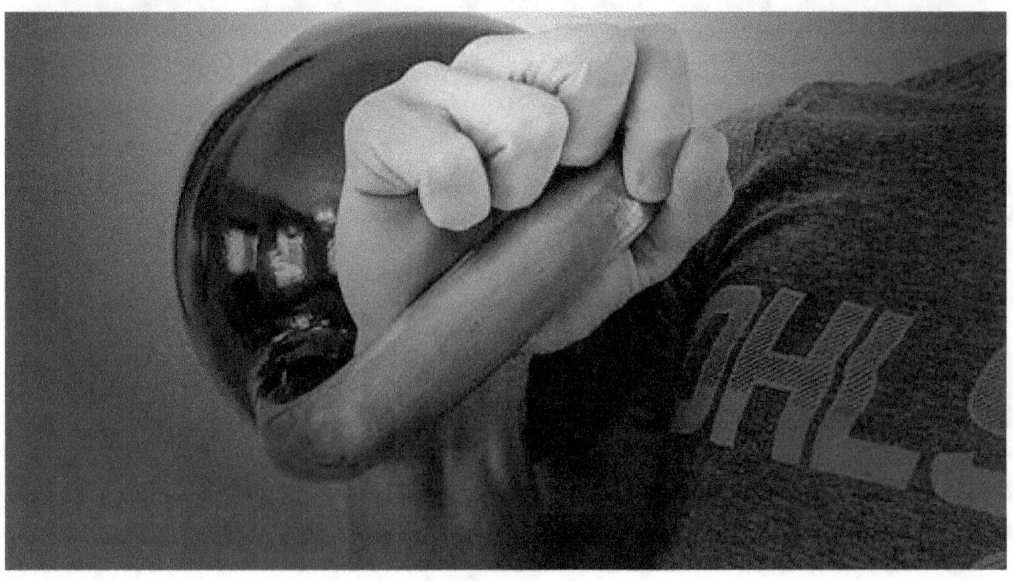

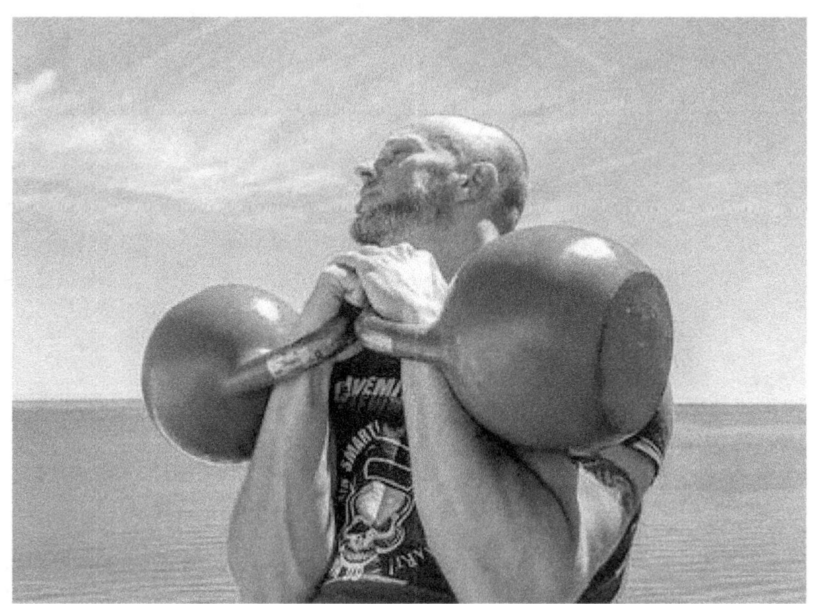

*Racking safety grip*

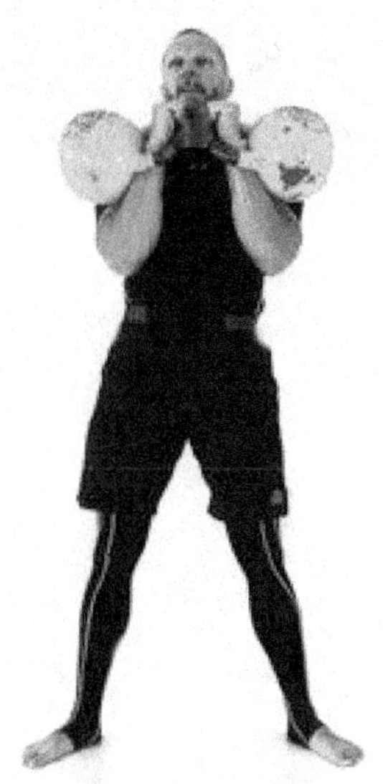 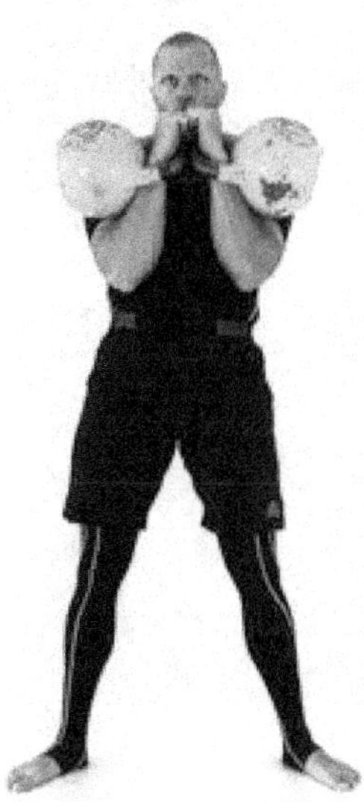

## Flat Hand Grip

The hand is flat or straight with all fingers pointing up and the thumb is around the horn. Can be employed for safety with two kettlebells, racking or in overhead lock-out.

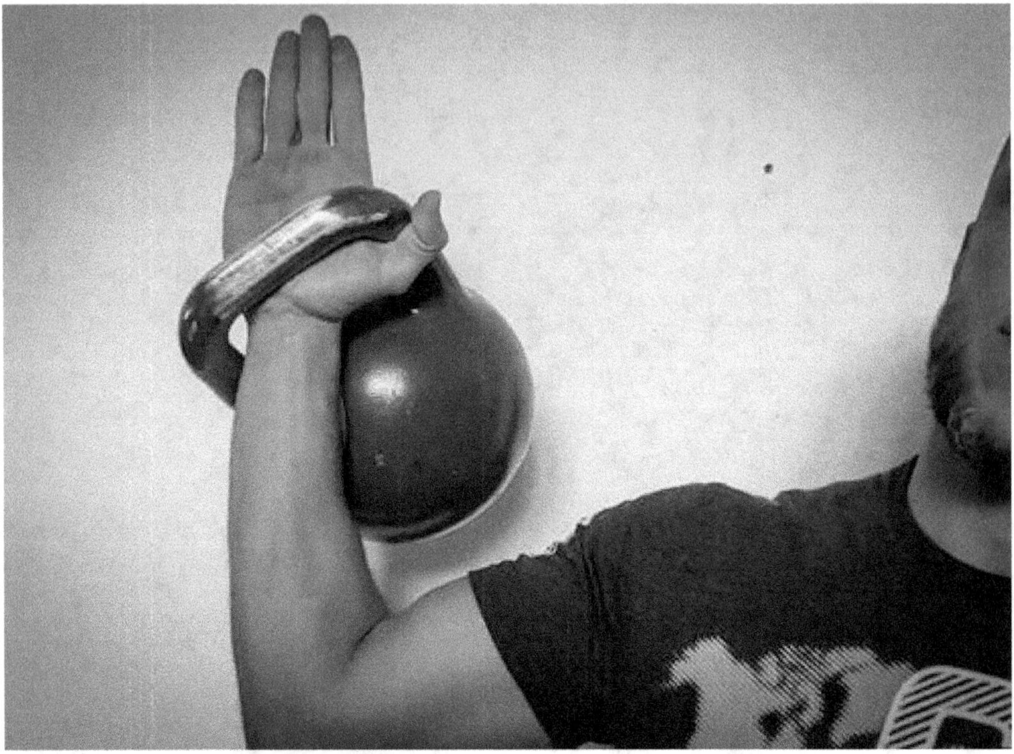

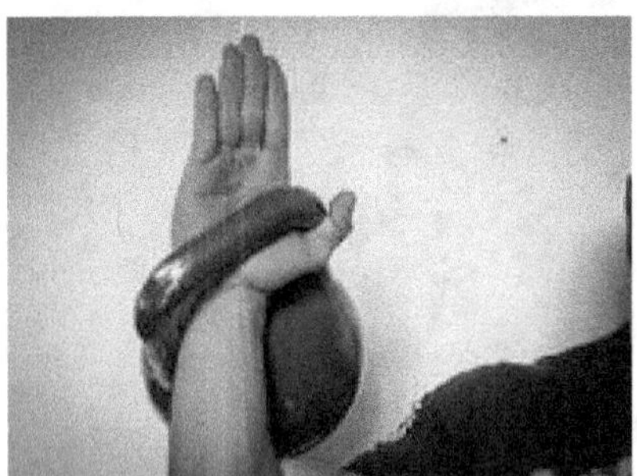

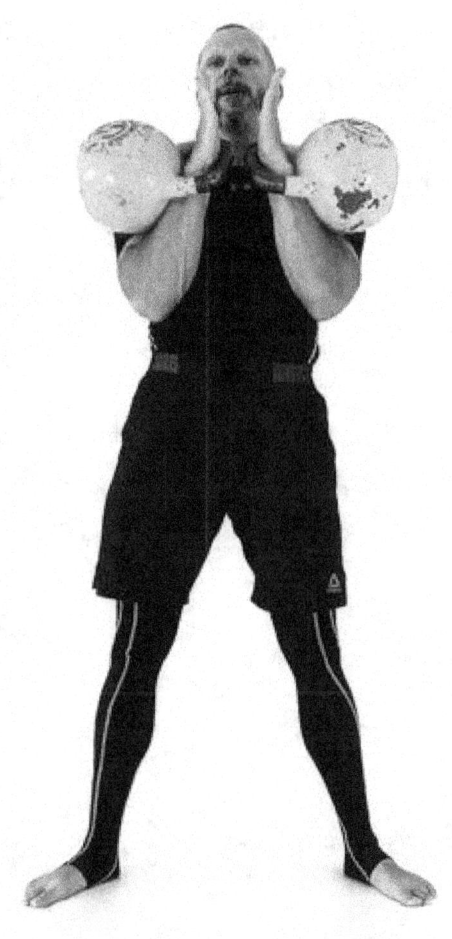

**Pinch Grip**

With this grip the thumb and fingers are used to pick up the kettlebell by the base of the kettlebell, this can only be performed with a smaller classic kettlebell. Used for working grip strength.

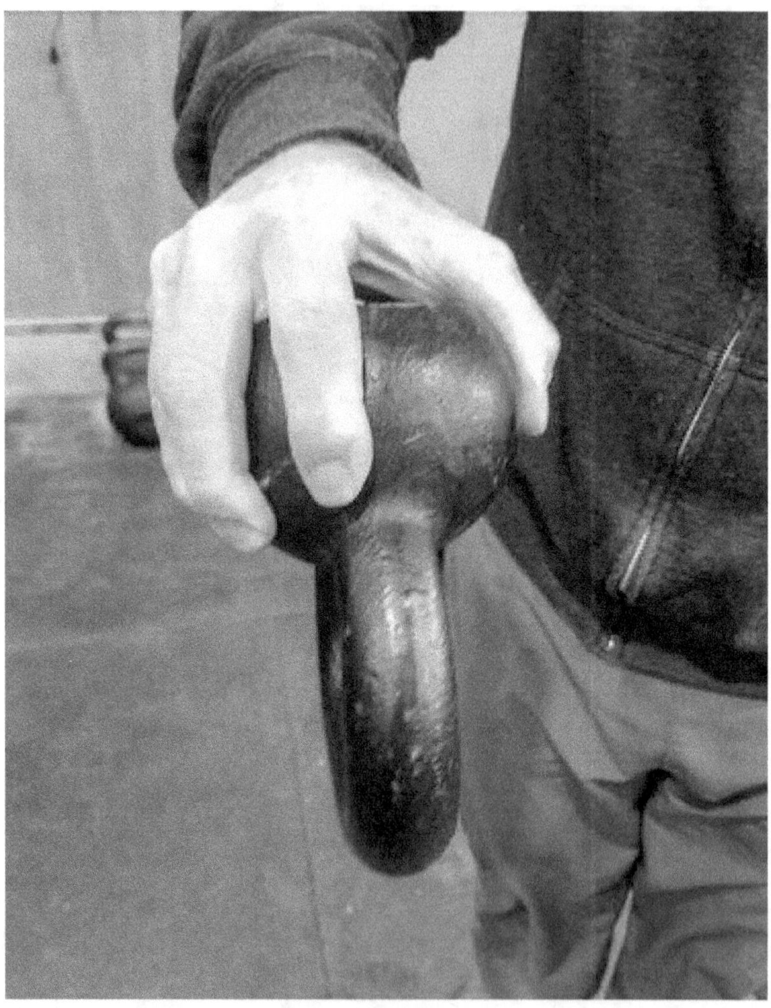

Photo provided by Robert Gagnon SFG II
www.RobGagnon.com

## Farmer Grip

**Grip:** middle of the handle.

**Handle:** one hand, four fingers and thumb locking the index finger down, or both the index and middle finger

**Ideal for:** farmer walks, suitcase dead lifts

With this grip, the hand is placed in the middle of the handle, and used when carrying a heavy Kettlebell beside the body with farmer walks or dead lifts. It should be noted that although the farmer walk grip is usually with a firm grip —contrary to most other grips— you can perform farmer walks with a hook grip as well to challenge the fingers more.

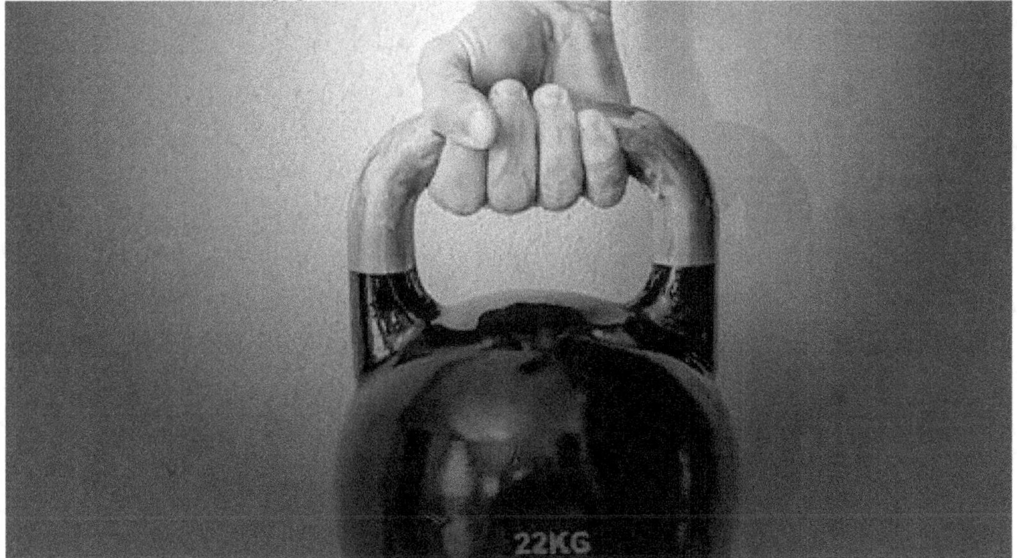


Farmer walks in action: https://www.youtube.com/watch?v=jqs8NGg50C0

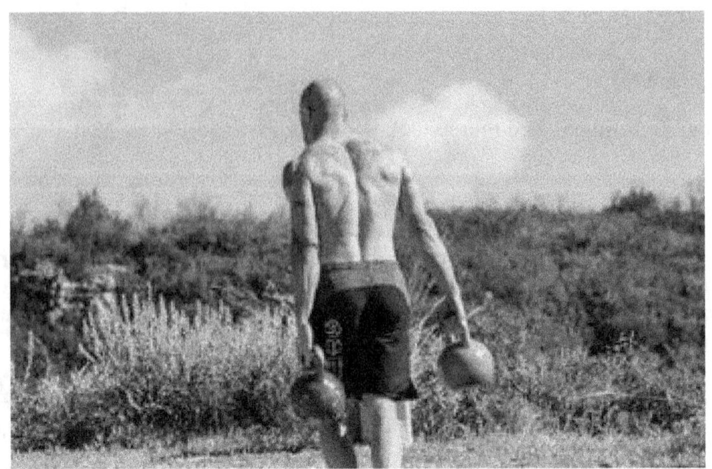

*Farmer walks near Barranco Blanco on the Costa del Sol*

## Tip of the Fingers Grip AKA Gorilla Grip

**Grip:** tip of the fingers.

**Handle:** the handle lays in the tips of the fingers which are shaped like when manicuring the finger nails.

**Ideal for:** farmer walks, suitcase dead lifts, dead lifts

This grip, is an awesome grip to work on grip strength, I personally started using this to improve my grip strength for BJJ (martial art) and baptised it the Gorilla Grip. The handle should nearly be falling of the fingers that's how little grip should be used. The thumb is not used, just the four finger tips.

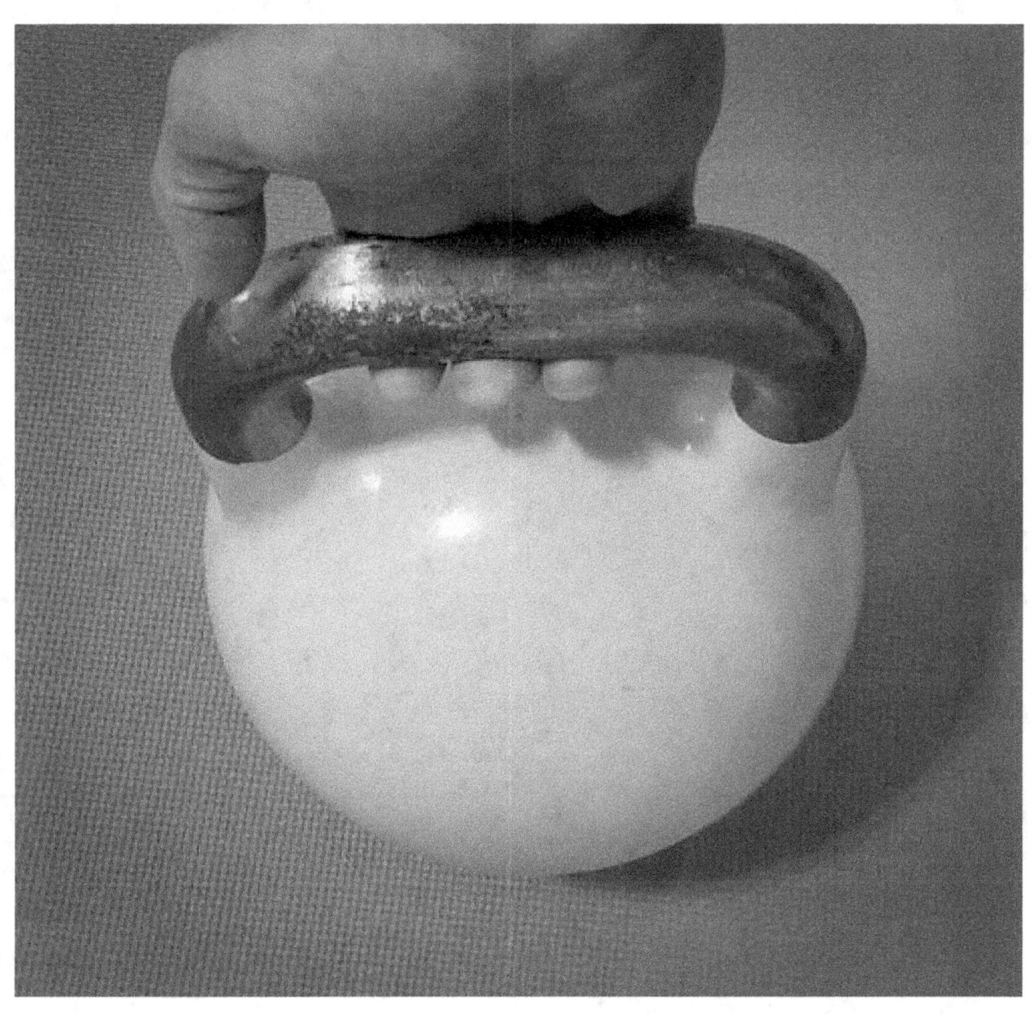

## Bottoms Up Grip

**Handle:** one hand, four fingers and thumb crushing the handle

**Ideal for:** bottoms up press, bottoms up squat

This grip is performed with a strong and firm grip on the handle while the Kettlebell is upside down, and used for bottoms up press or bottoms up Turkish get-up. The bottoms-up grip is great to work on grip strength and stability.

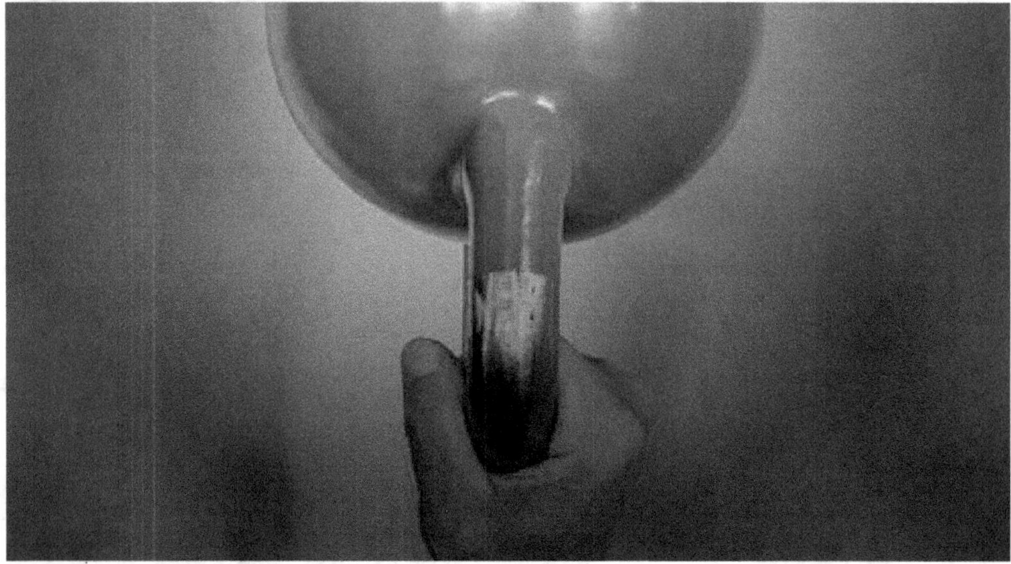

## Horn Grip

**Handle:** two hands, four fingers and thumb locking the index finger down on the horns

**Ideal for:** curls, lunge and twist, halo's

This grip is performed with both hands holding the horns, and is used for doing halo's and bicep curls.

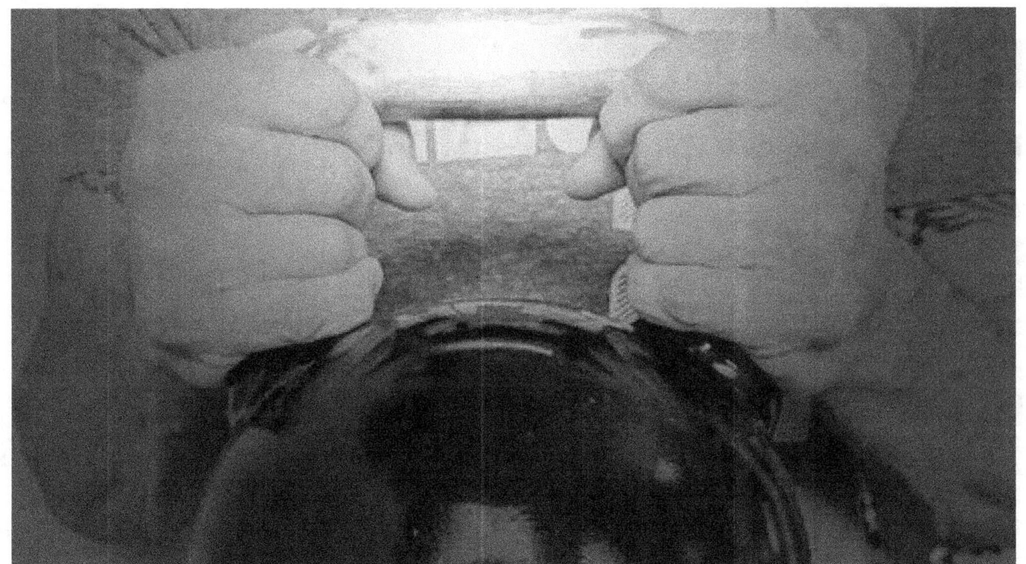

Russian twist in action: https://www.youtube.com/watch?v=_KbZno3KZdY

## Horn Grip Upside Down

**Handle:** two hands, four fingers and thumb locking the index finger down on the horns

**Ideal for:** Russian twists, pull overs, halo's

This grip is performed with the hands holding the horns while the kettlebell is upside down, and can be used for pull-overs and Russian twists.

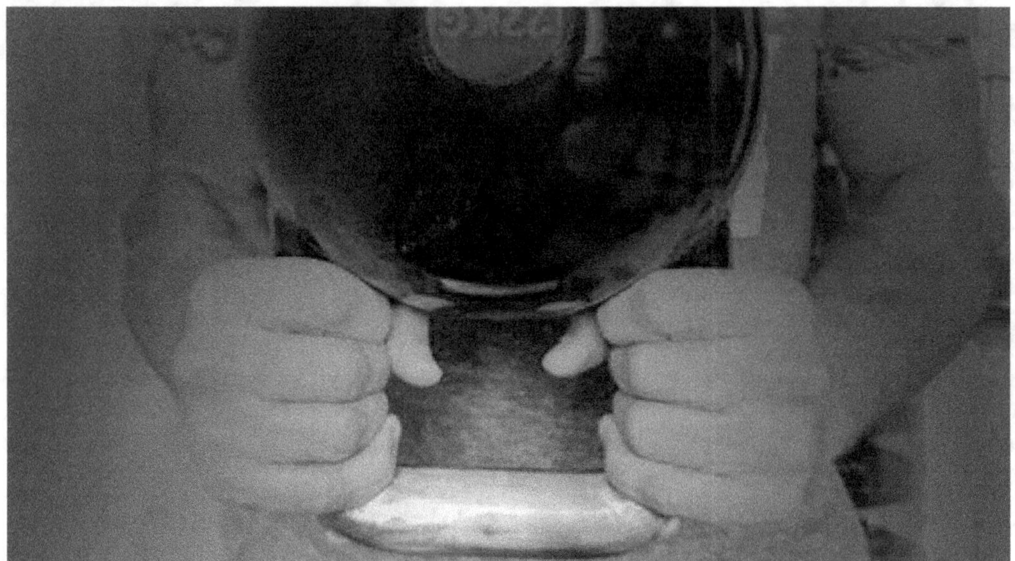

This is also a great grip to work on wrist strength with lateral wrist movement, you can do this in the air with a light bell or have the handle resting on the ground with a heavier bell. When resting the handle on the ground and base is up, the objective is to slowly move the bell forward to where it almost touches the ground, slowly and controlled bringing it back towards you as far as possible.

If you do this drill in the air it also works your biceps as you need to hold the forearms just above horizontal in a static position while moving the wrists. Of course, this will also require you to activate your lats, chest, back and abdominal muscles to provide a solid base where to perform this drill from.

                    Kettlebell Exercise Encyclopedia VOL. 4                    Taco Fleur

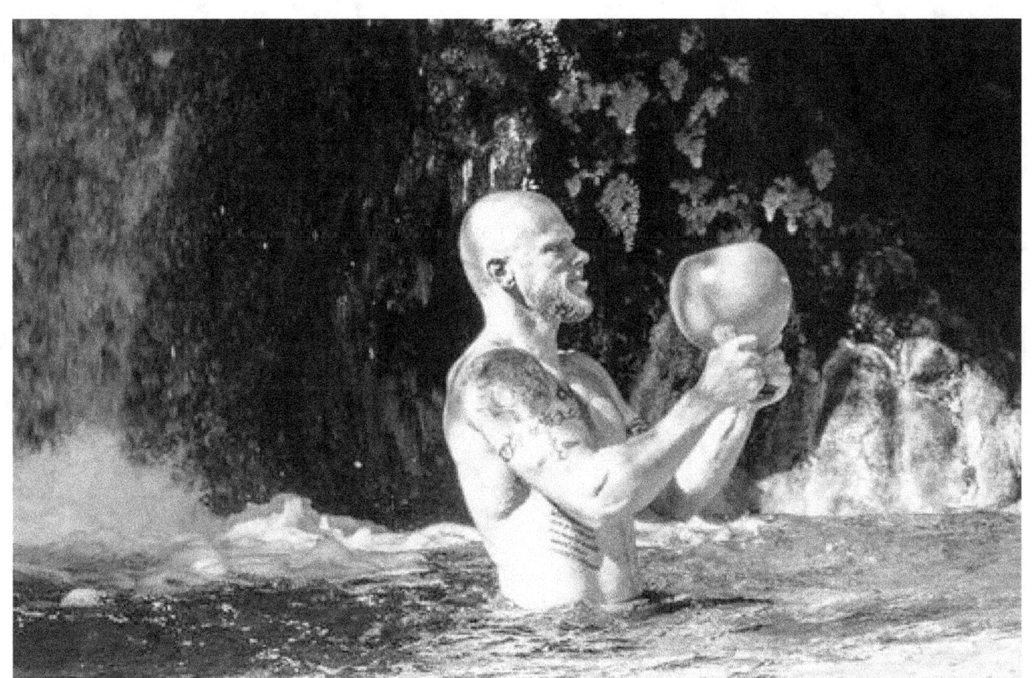

## Corner Grip

**Handle:** one hand, four fingers and thumb loose or locking the index finger down

**Ideal for:** around the body, figure eight

This grip is performed with the hand holding the handle in the corner, i.e. where the handle and horn intersects, used for around the body and figure eight's. A corner grip is mostly employed for passing the kettlebell to the other hand, whether you're juggling or switching arms.

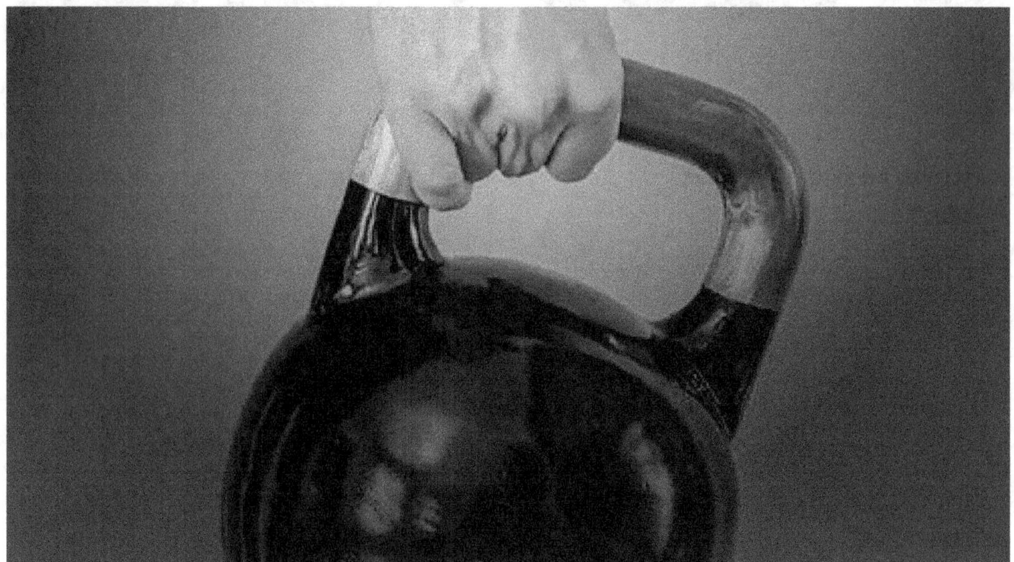

Corner grips with or without a finger lock like demonstrated in the following photo can also be used for single arm swings and snatches. Having your hand positioned there means it's already where it needs to end up in overhead position.

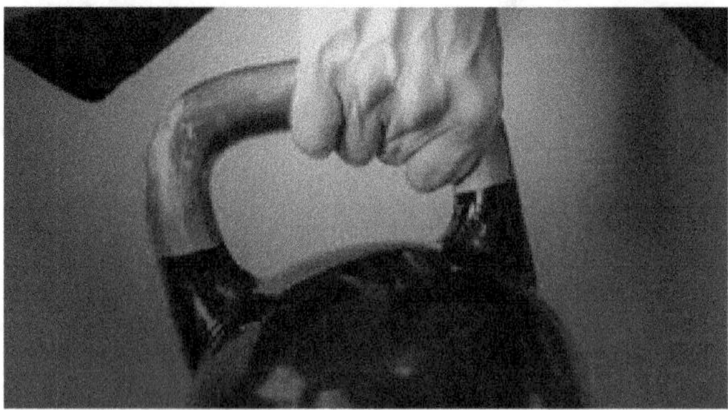

## Open Hand Horn Grip

**Handle:** two hands, all fingers slightly squeezing the bell and the thumbs folded around the bottom of the horns

**Ideal for:** laying down chest presses, front squats, skull crushers

With this grip both hands are used, palms are open and slightly squeezing the bell which is resting within the palms, the thumbs are folded around the bottom of the horns. This grip is used for front squats and skull crushers.

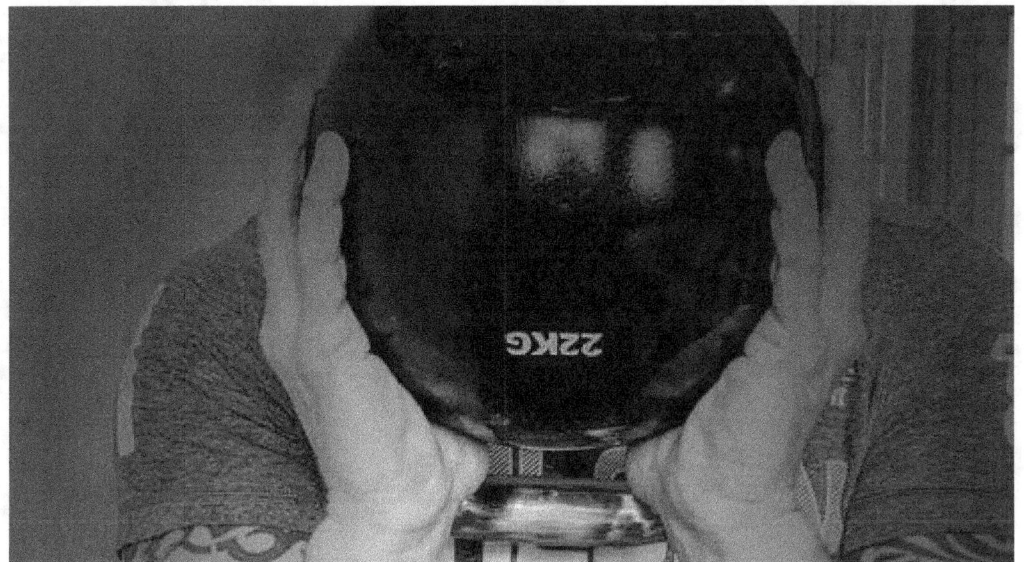

## Loose Grip

**Handle:** one hand, four fingers and thumb loosely around the handle

**Ideal for:** any press variation, any overhead work, racking

This grip is performed by keeping your fingers loose rather than tightly closed and squeezing, it's used for the overhead position like presses and snatches.

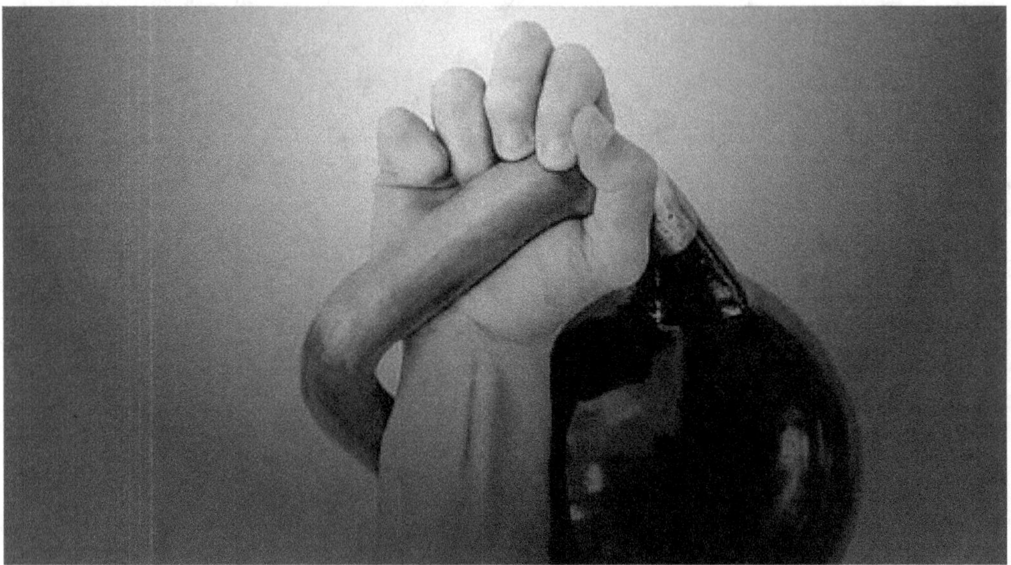

A great analogy to get the idea across for CrossFitters is thinking about a false grip.

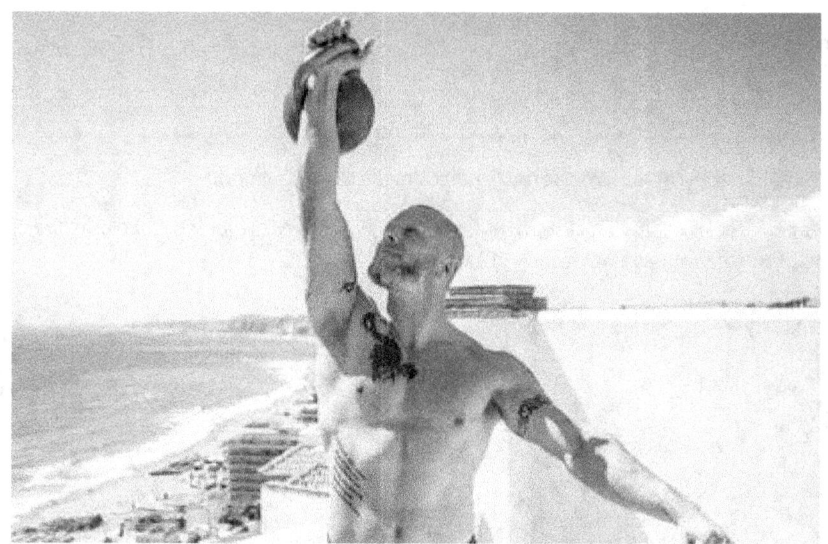

## Interlocking Grip

**Handle:** two hands, all fingers interlocking and thumb through the corners

**Ideal for:** racking rest, anything performed with a rack, front squats

This grip is performed by interlocking the fingers of both hands, elbows tight into the side of the body, and is used for front squats or racked lunges.

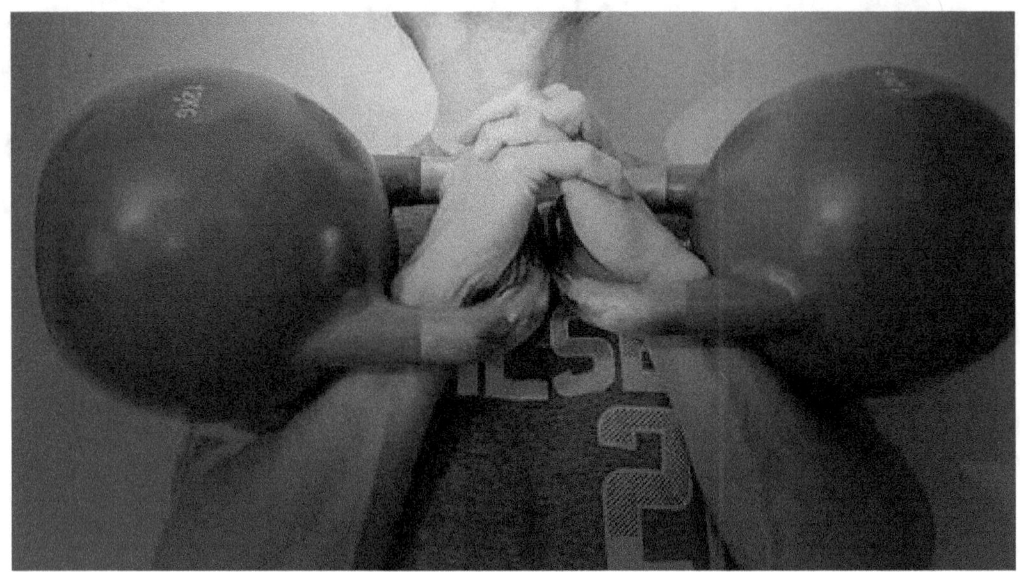

## Stacking Grip

**Handle:** two hands, several fingers holding on to the handle of the stacked kettlebell

**Ideal for:** racking rest, anything going rack to overhead

This grip is performed by placing the handles on top of each other and several fingers holding on to the second handle while the top hand is over the bottom hand, used for resting or anything going overhead like the press, push press or jerk.

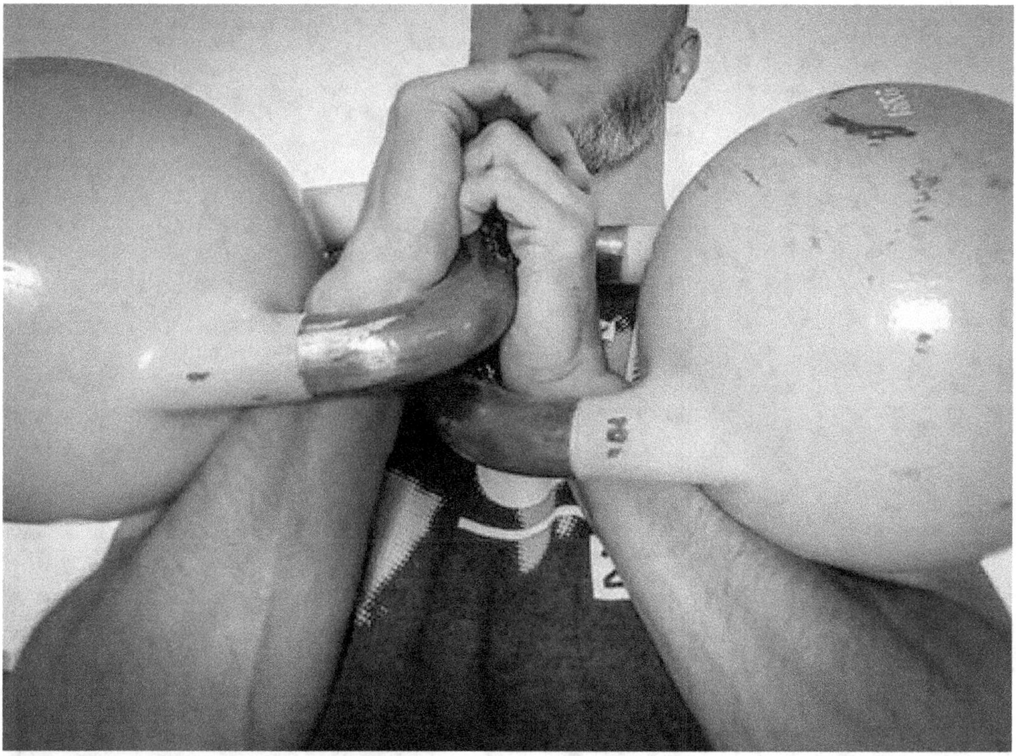

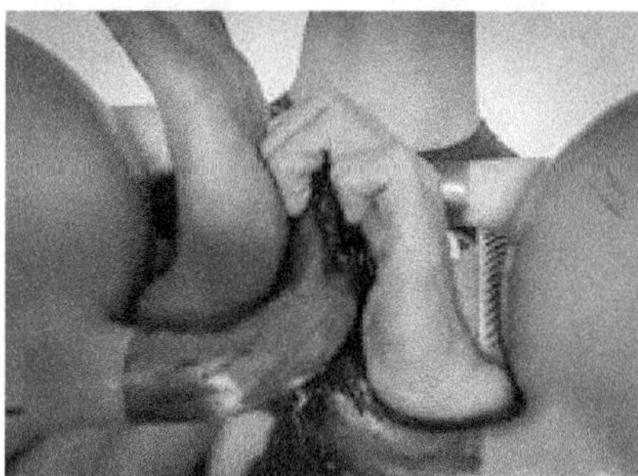

## Open Palm Grip

**Handle:** handle is resting against the underside of the forearm

**Ideal for:** increasing difficulty of presses

This grip is performed with the bell resting in the open palm and handle against the underside of the forearm. Great for working on wrist strength.

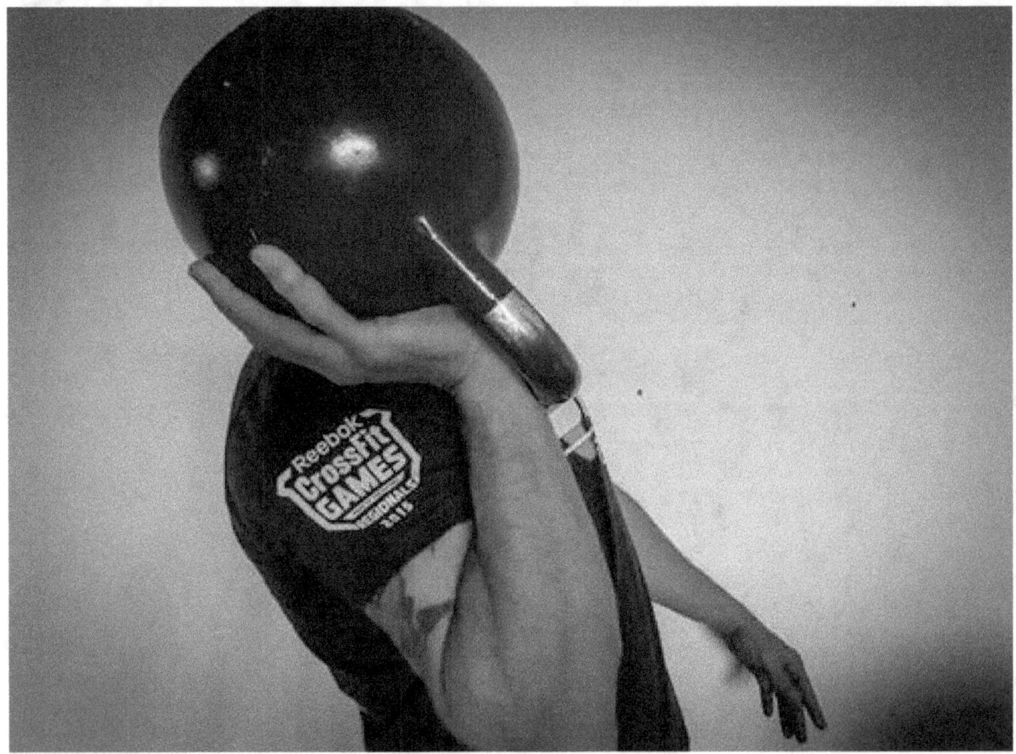

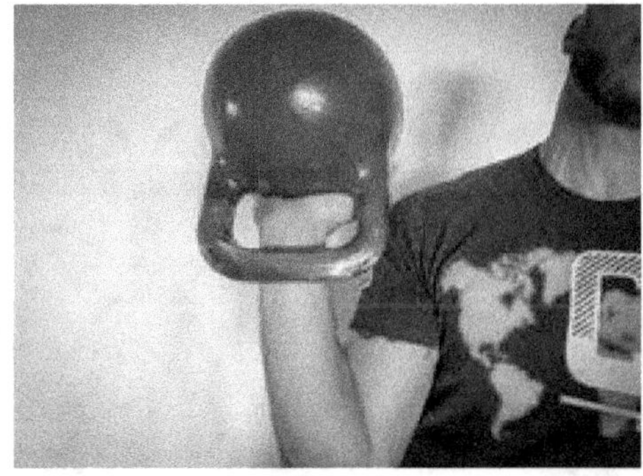

Open palm snatch in action: go.cavemantraining.com/kbe-vid-136

## Waiters Grip

**Handle:** the handle does not come into play

**Ideal for:** increasing difficulty of presses

This grip is performed with the base resting on the open palm. Great for working on wrist strength. This grip is named for obvious reasons, the way the kettlebell rests on the palm resembles that of a waiter carrying a tray.

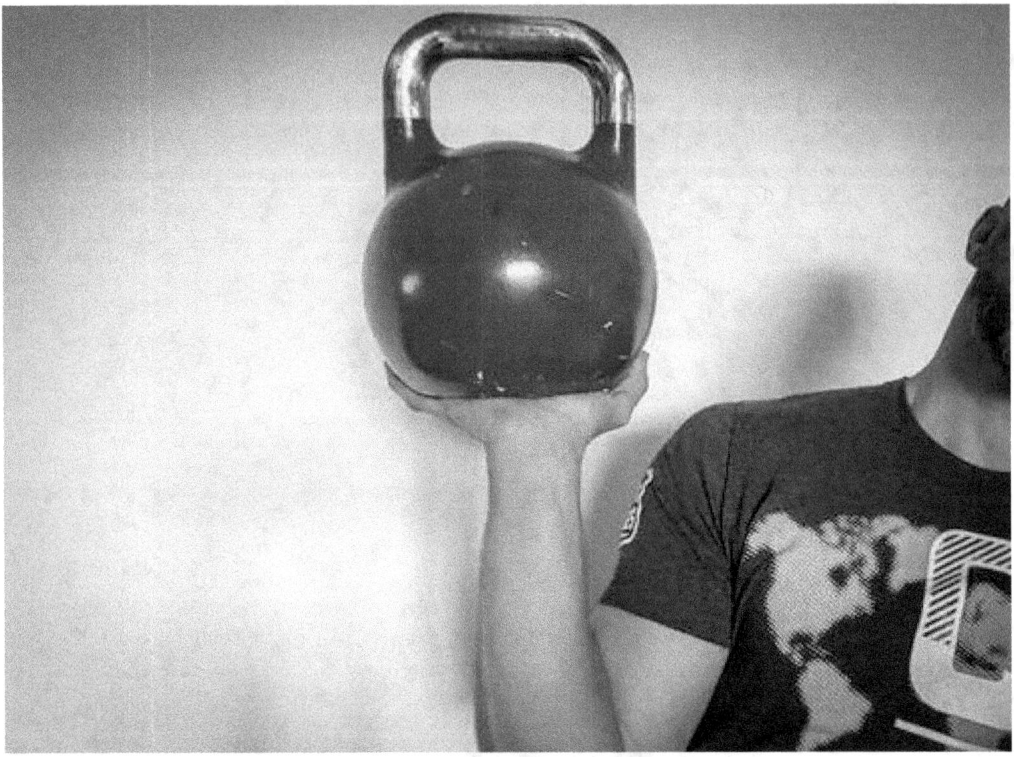

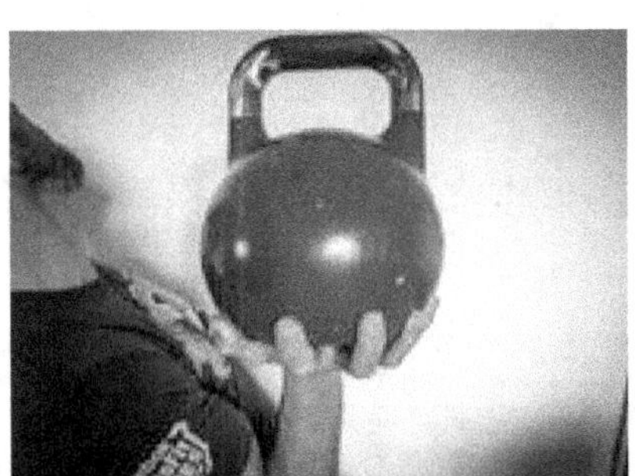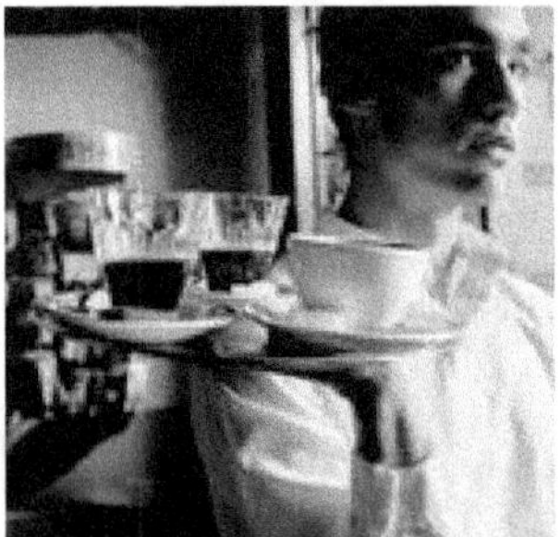

*Illustrated is the waiters grip from different angle and a waiter carrying a tray*

Once you get into kettlebell juggling you can swing and catch the kettlebell directly into waiters grip, from there you can perform an overhead squat. This variation requires a more explosive swing to get the kettlebell high and flip into waiters grip.

You can see the waiters grip in action here: go.cavemantraining.com/kbe-vid-137

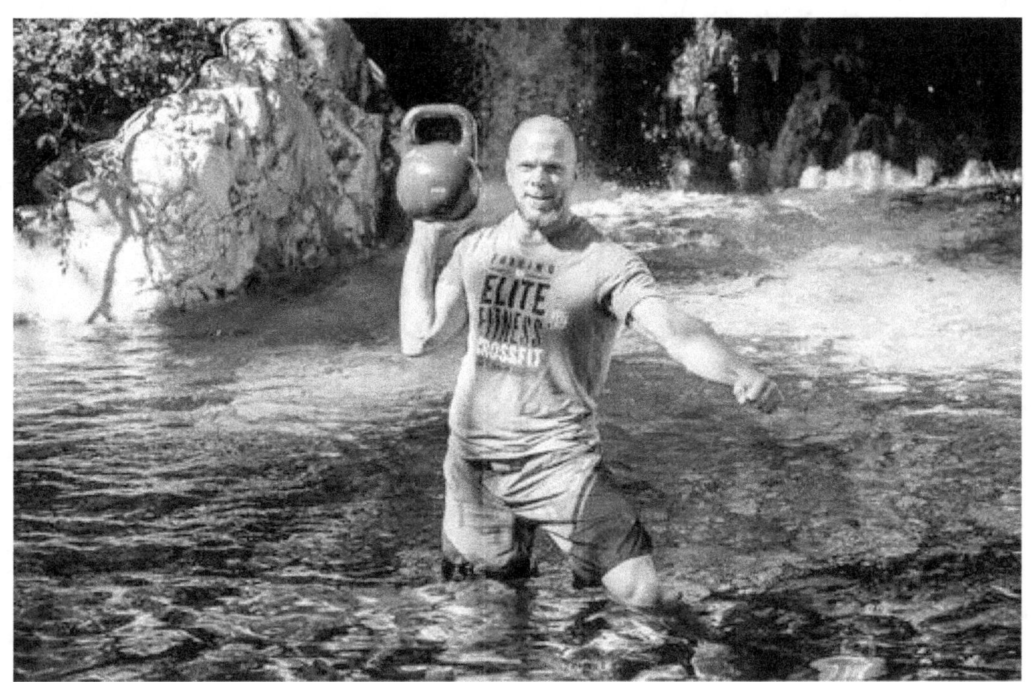

## Goblet Grip

**Handle:** the handle does not come into play

**Ideal for:** front-squat

This grip is performed with the palms pressing around the bell, the handle is up or down. The grip is named for obvious reasons, the shape of the kettlebell with handle down resembles that of a goblet. With the handle facing up this grip is called the *reverse goblet grip*. The higher you go up the bell with your palms, the harder you need to squeeze, palms towards the bottom and the bell is resting more within the palms.

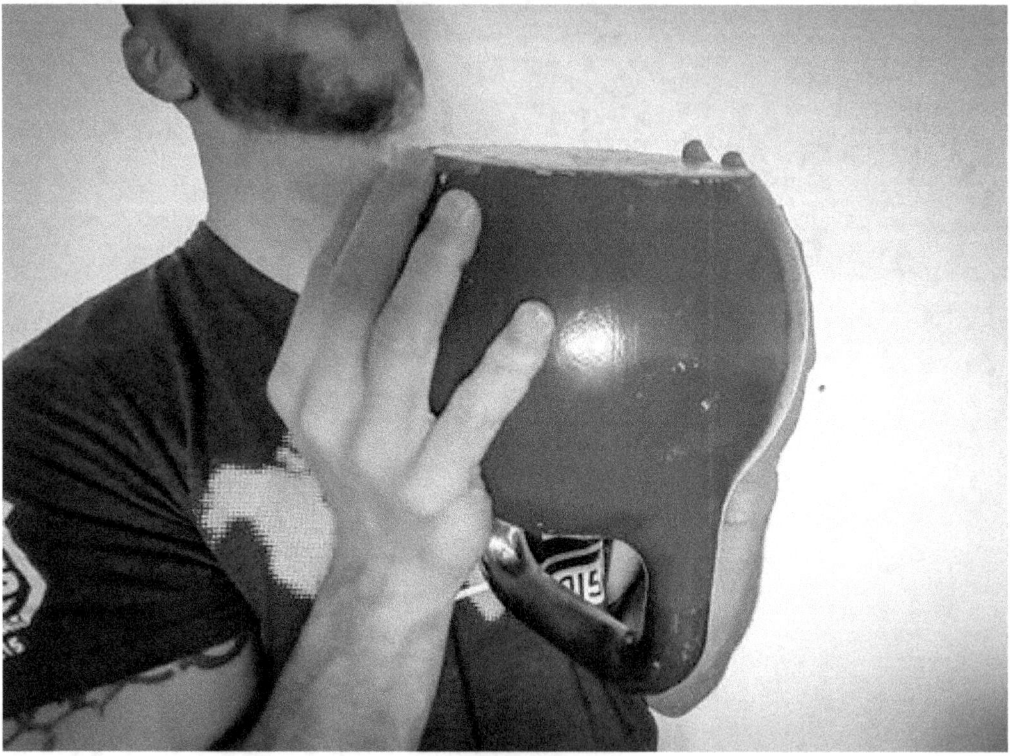

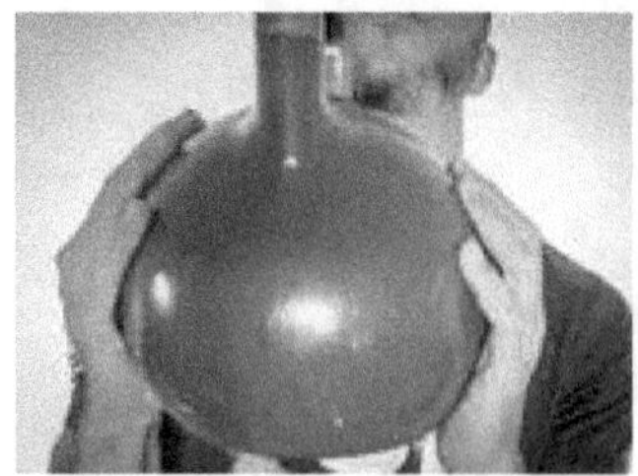

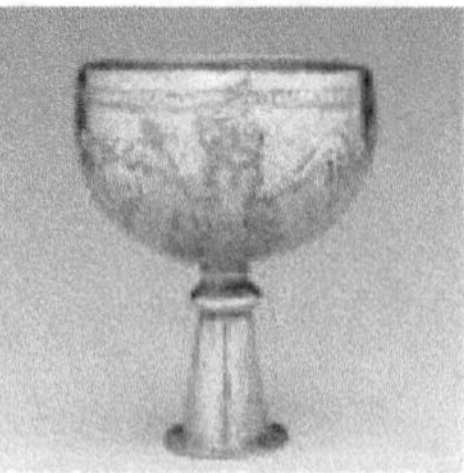

You can watch a video demonstrating the *goblet grip* in a *goblet squat*.
go.cavemantraining.com/kbe-vid-138

## Crush Grip

**Handle:** the handle does not come into play

**Ideal for:** front-squat, static hold, push-up

This grip is performed with the palms crushing the bell, the handle is up or down. Similar to the goblet grip but more crushing with the palms. Great for working the pectoralis.

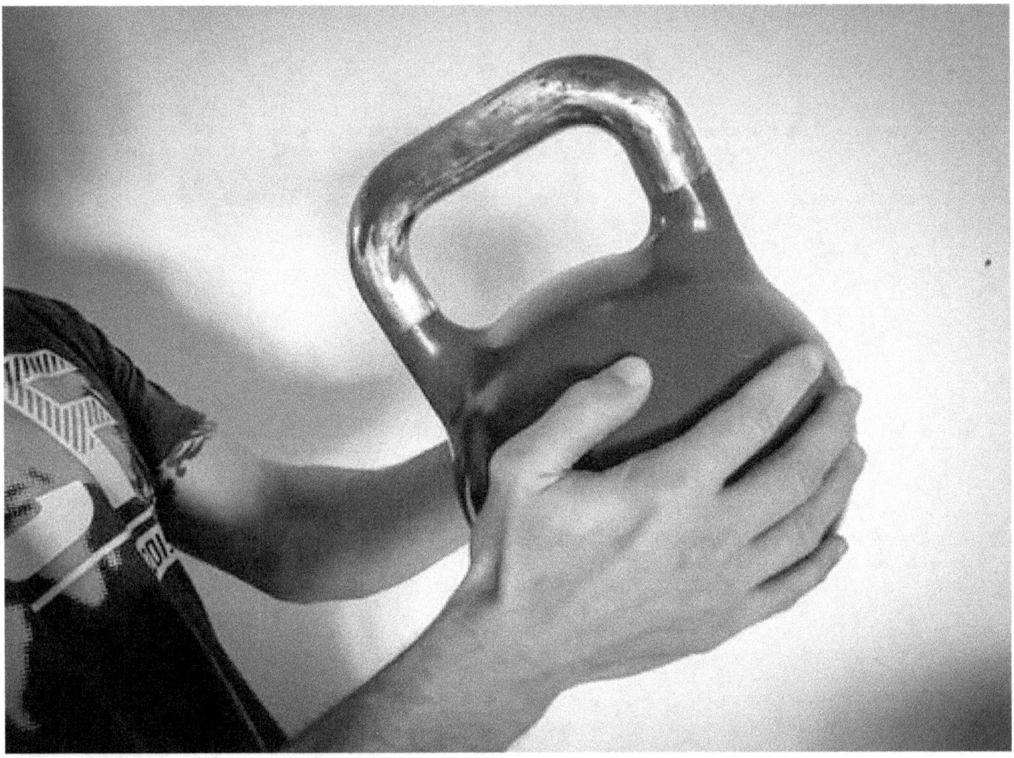

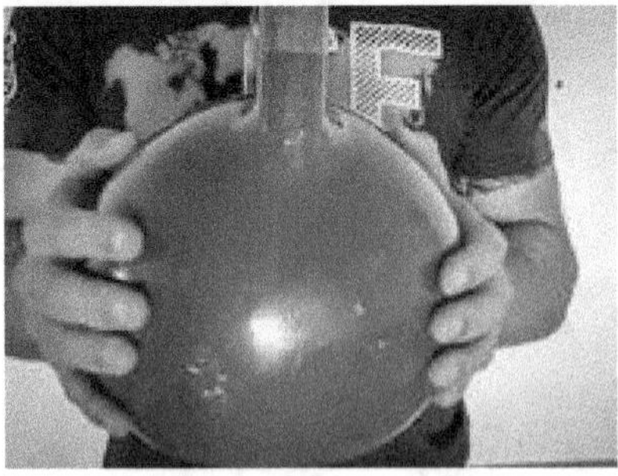

Have you tried the *kettlebell crush push-up* yet?

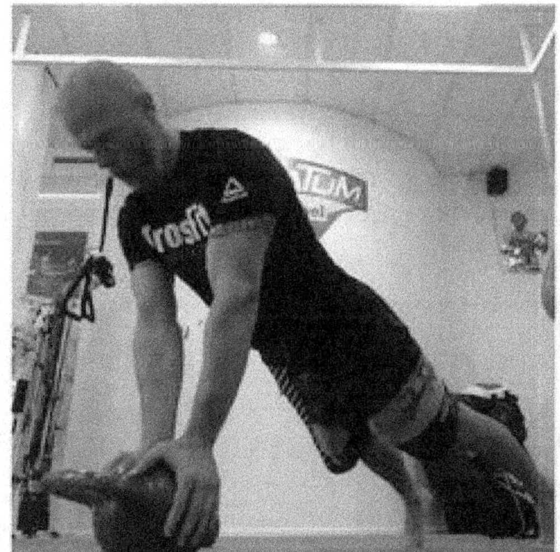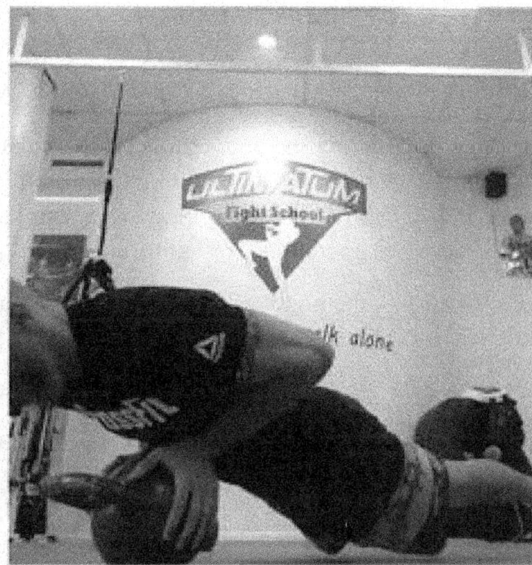

You can watch a short video here: go.cavemantraining.com/kbe-vid-139

## Thumb Grip (AKA Noob Grip)

**Handle:** the handle is resting more on the heel of the thumb than with the loose grip.

**Ideal for:** press

The bell rests on the inside of the arm, complete opposite of the loose grip, the handle is resting more on the heel of the thumb. Great for shifting the weight from the outside of the arm to the inside. Full range reps from racking are not possible with this grip. Try this one with the side press starting above the shoulder and returning above the shoulder.

I like to call this the noob grip as this is the grip a lot of new people use the first ever time they lift a kettlebell without instruction.

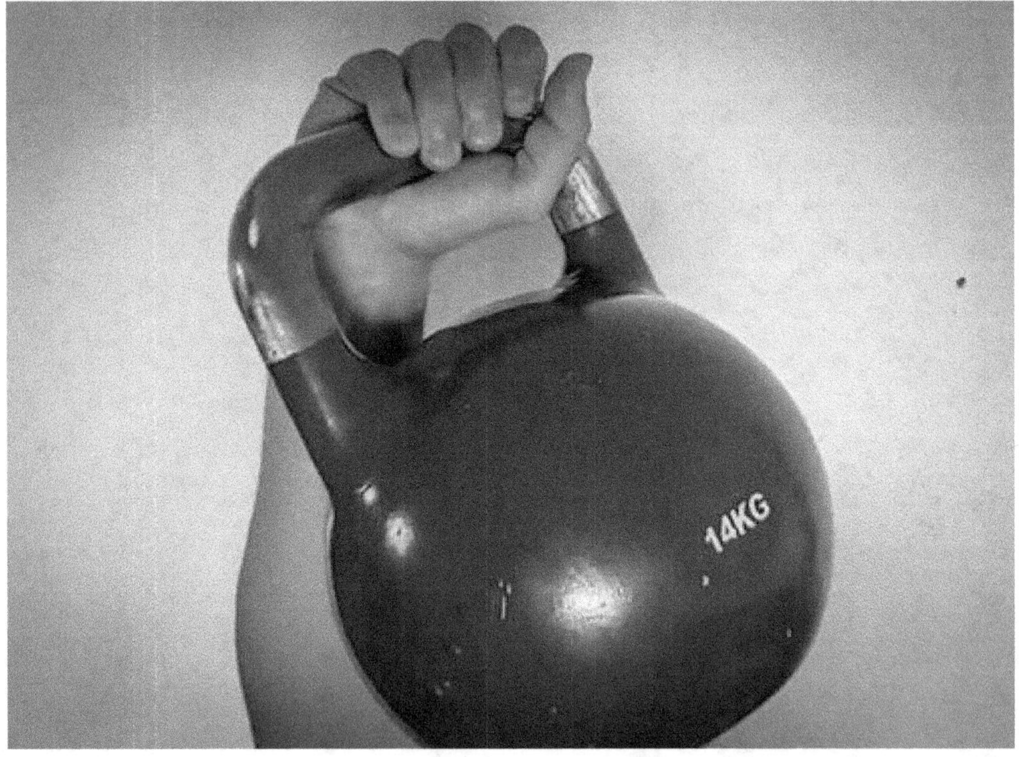


Find out why I named this the *noob grip* and why it's such a great grip to employ after you learned all other grips. www.cavemantraining.com/caveman-kettlebells/24-unconventional-kettlebell-exercises-three-broken/

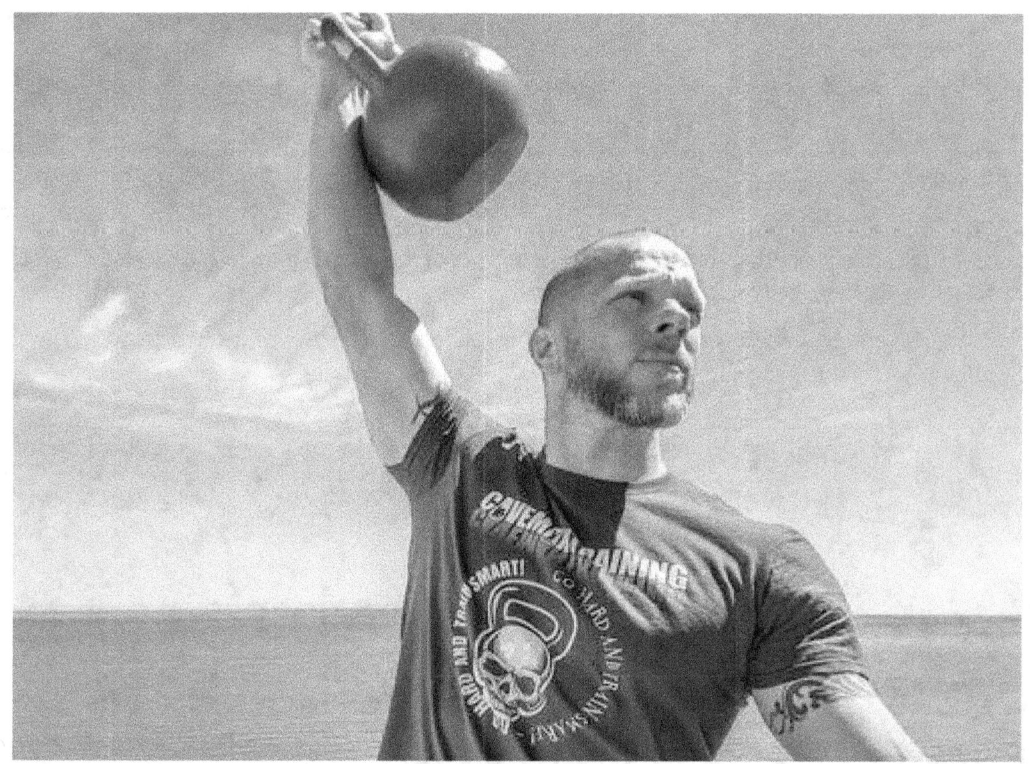

*Noob grip press*

More info about the *noob grip squat* can be found here www.cavemantraining.com/caveman-kettlebells/even-kettlebell-squat-bro/

Check out the combination of noob grip squat and press, try it yourself and notice the instability it provides, which is great once you've gained some strength and technique by implementing common grips. go.cavemantraining.com/kbe-vid-140

## Fireman's Grip

This grip is solely used for carrying the kettlebells on or over the shoulders and is what I call the fireman's grip due to the close resemblance of the fireman's carry. With this grip your hand is holding the handle in the middle and is resting more in the fingers, the elbows are up and the kettlebell is resting on or over your shoulder. Can be performed with one or two kettlebells, one on each side.

Great for back squats, i.e. the weight is resting on the back rather than the front, can also be used for just carrying the kettlebells and walking.

Watch a demonstration of the Fireman's Squat in the following video go.cavemantraining.com/kbe-vid-141

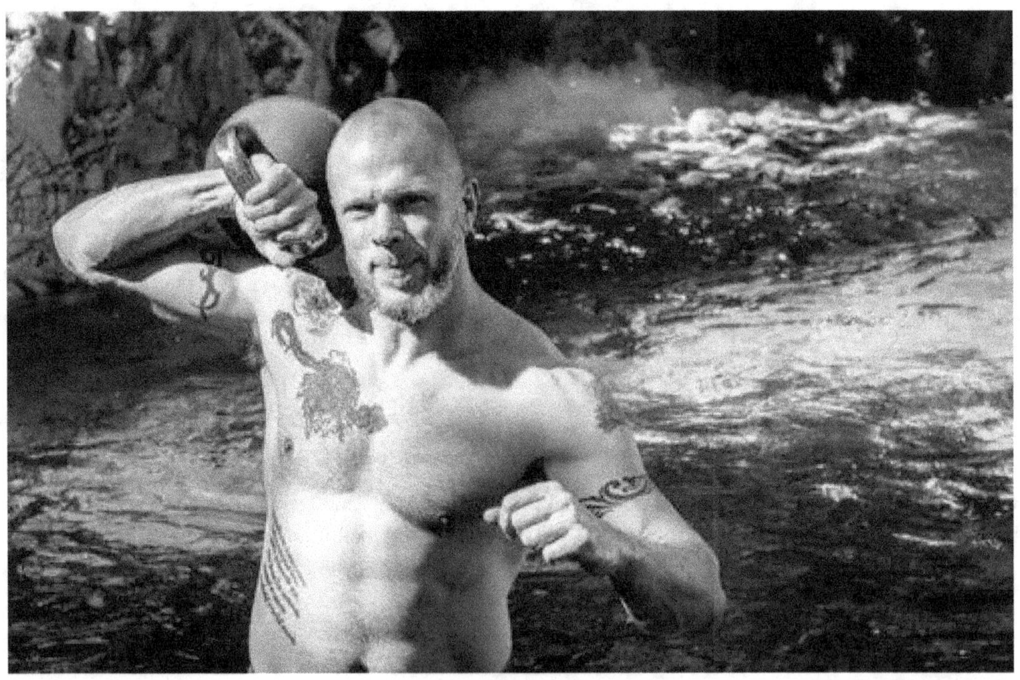

## Stacked Grip

This grip is used to work with **multiple** kettlebells in one hand. It's a great grip to add more weight to your deadlifts or overhead work. The grip requires a lot more grip strength as well, as double or triple handles/weight will require more grip strength.

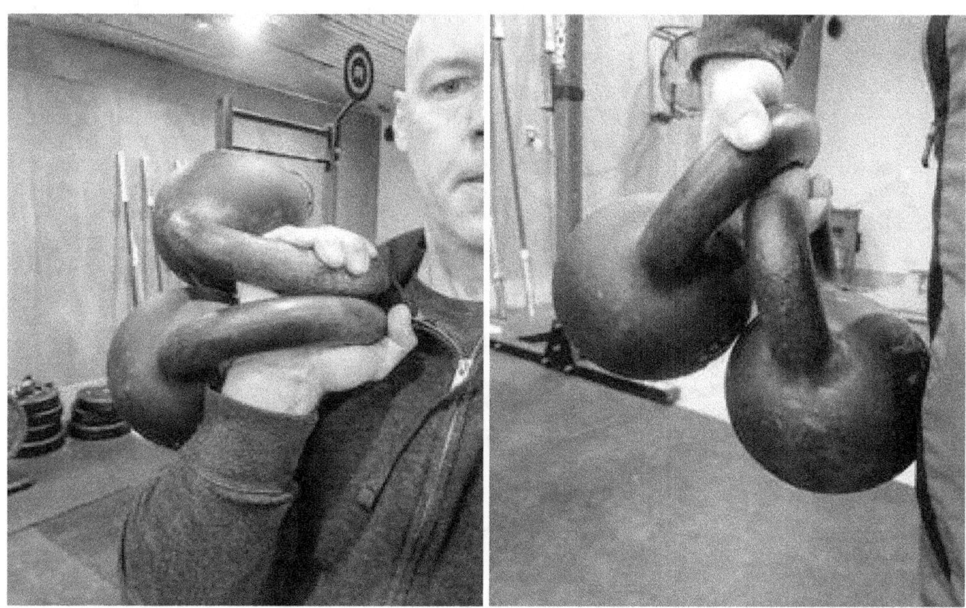

Photo provided by Robert Gagnon SFG II
www.RobGagnon.com

**NOTE**
If you experience forearm bruising, tenderness or pain from bell pressure, make sure you check out my detailed article on this topic, you won't find anything more detailed and intricate about this issue elsewhere. Search Google for 'Cavemantraining forearm pressure, bruising and pain'.

# Other Kettlebell/Fitness Books

Other kettlebell books by Cavemantraining are:
* Kettlebell Guide For Beginners
* Kettlebell Training Fundamentals
* Kettlebell Training Fundamentals (Spanish)
* Master The Hip Hinge
* Master The Basic Kettlebell Swing
* Master The Kettlebell Clean
* Master The Kettlebell Press
* Kettlebell Workouts And Challenges 1.0
* Kettlebell Workouts And Challenges 2.0
* Kettlebell Strength Program Prometheus
* Snatch Physics
* Kettlebells For Mobility And Flexibility
* Caveman Mobility Program
* Flexibility, Mobility, And Strength Without Yoga

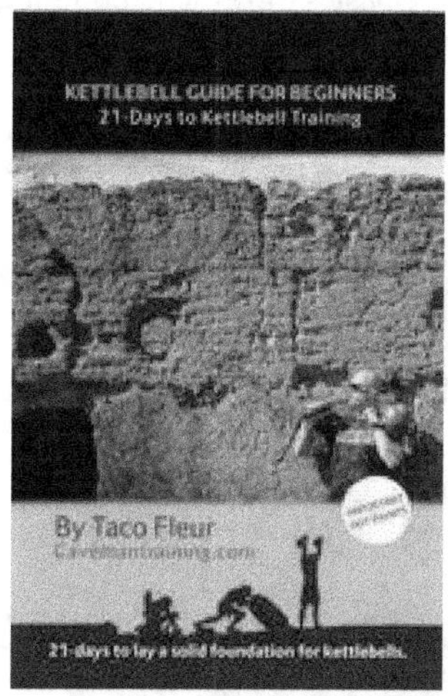


This kettlebell training book is a quick introduction to kettlebell training for beginners with dot points rather than lengthy explanations.
**Buy on Amazon** go.cavemantraining.com/amazon-1
**Prime Video** go.cavemantraining.com/amazon-2
**DVD** go.cavemantraining.com/amazon-3
**Blu-ray** go.cavemantraining.com/amazon-4
**Udemy course** go.cavemantraining.com/udemy-1

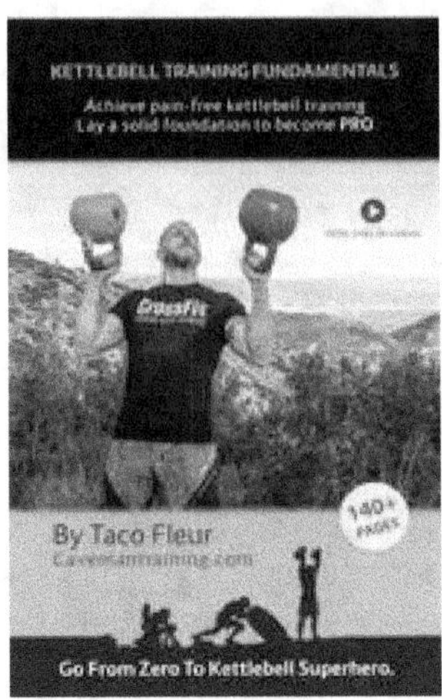

If you're looking to get into kettlebell training then there is no better book than Kettlebell Training Fundamentals, one of the best books for kettlebell training beginners to pick up and lay the proper foundations for a lifelong kettlebell journey. If you want to progress in kettlebell training then you need to master the basics, these are the basics of kettlebell training and they take you step-by-step to where you want to be, performing the fundamentals movements of kettlebell training safely and effectively. **Buy on Amazon**. go.cavemantraining.com/amazon-5
**Direct download**. go.cavemantraining.com/download-1

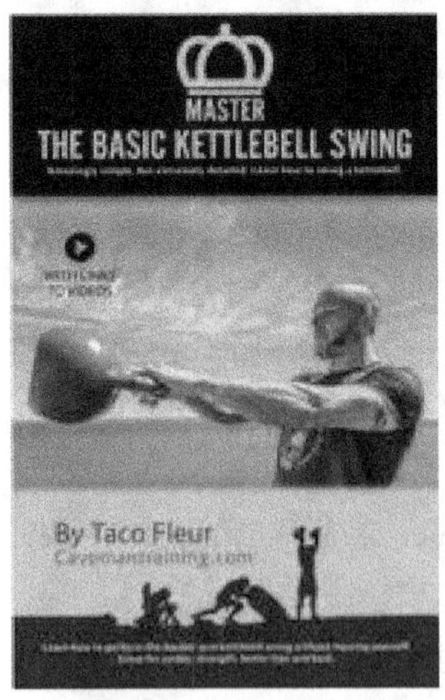

This book is your first step to becoming a serious kettlebell trainer or kettlebell enthusiast. Improve your cardiovascular endurance and potentially irradiate neck and back pain with one simple exercise. If you're a Crossfitter and want to get more efficient at snatching and the American Swing, then learn the foundation for both, the conventional kettlebell swing AKA Russian Swing. **Buy on Amazon**. go.cavemantraining.com/amazon-6
**Direct download**. go.cavemantraining.com/download-2

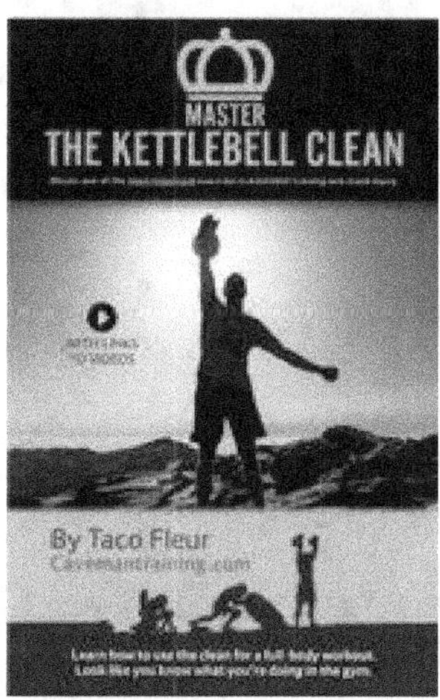

If you want to get into kettlebell training, you can't go past the clean, as simple as this exercise might sound, there is a whole lot involved, and is usually an area in which beginners get injured. I will cover most common injuries and how to avoid them.
**Buy on Amazon**. go.cavemantraining.com/amazon-7
**Direct download**. go.cavemantraining.com/download-3

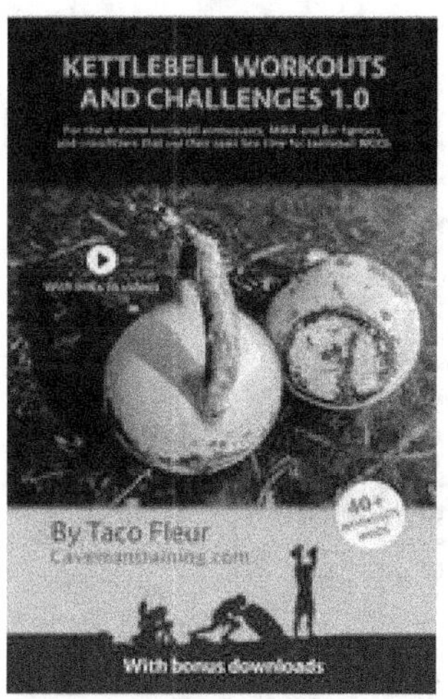

40+ serious kettlebell workouts, 4 kettlebell challenges, many are paired with very detailed videos.
**Buy on Amazon**. go.cavemantraining.com/amazon-8
**Direct download**. go.cavemantraining.com/download-4

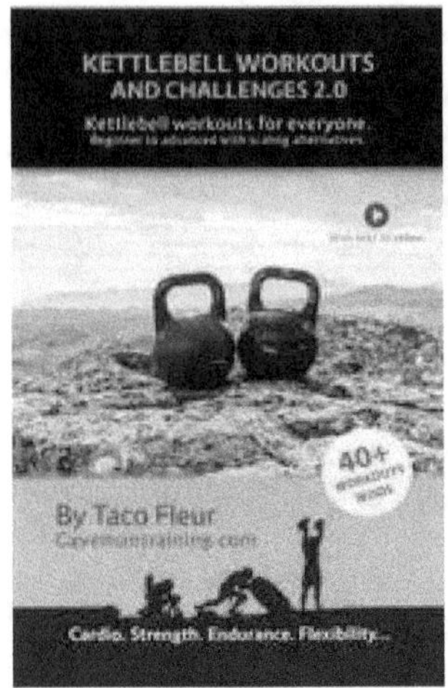

This book is targeted to at-home kettlebell enthusiasts, MMA and BJJ fighters, and crossfitters that use their open box time for kettlebell WODs. This book is even for budding trainers who want to know more about the Cavemantraining programs, and learn the basics on how to run them.  40+ serious kettlebell workouts and several kettlebell challenges, many paired with very detailed videos.
**Buy on Amazon**. go.cavemantraining.com/amazon-9
**Direct download**. go.cavemantraining.com/download-5

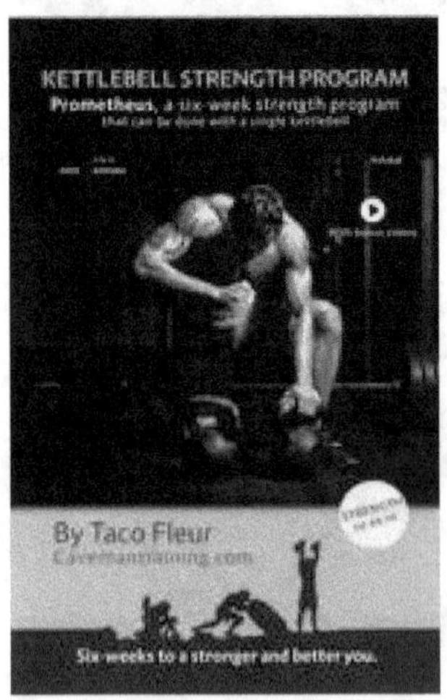

A six-week kettlebell strength program that can be completed with a single kettlebell. The program is simple and based on three super-powerful kettlebell exercises that work the full-body.
**Buy on Amazon**. go.cavemantraining.com/amazon-10
**Direct download**. go.cavemantraining.com/download-6

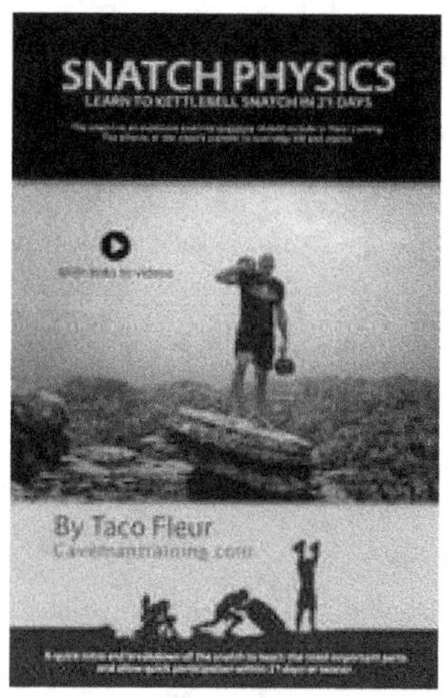

The kettlebell snatch is a full body exercise that delivers amazing effects. The snatch can be used to increase cardiovascular endurance, muscular endurance, strength, flexibility, core stability, explosive power, and much more. The snatch truly works each and every major joint in the body, ankles, knees, hips, shoulders, elbow, and wrists. For strength, you can't deny the major areas that will improve, such as, latissimus dorsi, deltoid, triceps, erector spinae, abdominals, glute, hamstrings, calves, hip flexors, quadriceps, lumbrical muscles, and many more.
**Buy on Amazon**. go.cavemantraining.com/amazon-11
**Direct download**. go.cavemantraining.com/download-7

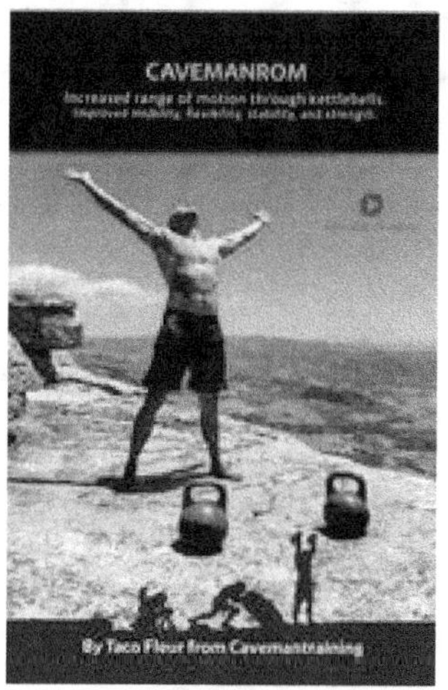

CAVEMANROM is all about loaded exercises for flexibility, stability, proprioception, strength, coordination, and everything else that increases mobility and range of motion. Injury-proof yourself. **Buy on Amazon**. go.cavemantraining.com/amazon-12

# Online Kettlebell Courses

- From Zero to Kettlebell Superhero in 4 Weeks (or less)
  www.udemy.com/from-zero-to-kettlebell-superhero — ~~$69.99~~
  With discount coupon: RCIL7W — **$15.99**

- 21-Days to Kettlebell Training for Beginners
  www.udemy.com/kettlebell-training-for-beginners — ~~$74.99~~
  With discount coupon: 5Z6P3V — **$14.99**

- Kettlebell Training **PREMIUM**
  www.udemy.com/kettlebell-training — ~~$149.99~~
  With discount coupon: C4DP41 — **$24.99**

- Beginner Kettlebells for Females (Authored by Anna Junghans)
  www.udemy.com/kettlebells-for-females — ~~$59.99~~
  With discount coupon: KRJO2E — **$14.99**

- Kettlebells—A VITAL Course to Take
  www.udemy.com/kettlebell-exercise — ~~$79.99~~
  With discount coupon: 98ZLUT — **$14.99**

- Kettlebells for Great Looking Shoulders
  www.udemy.com/kettlebells-for-shoulder-strength — ~~$39.99~~
  With discount coupon: RP8NYF — **$9.99**

- Kettlebell Exercise for Cardio and Weight Loss
  www.udemy.com/kettlebell-snatch/ — ~~$149.99~~
  With discount coupon: 59QI3O — **$29.99**

- Kettlebell Workouts
  www.udemy.com/kettlebell-workouts — ~~$74.95~~
  With discount coupon: WG7ILS — **$19.99**

# Online Kettlebell Certifications For Trainers

- Kettlebell Fundamentals Trainer L3.0
  www.cavemantraining.com/shop/training-course/kettlebell-fundamentals-trainer-l3-0/

- Kettlebell Snatch Trainer L3.0 + L4
  www.cavemantraining.com/shop/training-course/online-kettlebell-snatch-certification-by-cavemantraining/

- Kettlebell Clean Trainer L3.0 + L3.1
  www.cavemantraining.com/shop/training-course/kettlebell-clean-variations/

- CAVEMANROM Trainer L3.0
  www.cavemantraining.com/shop/certification/cavemanrom-trainer-online-certification/

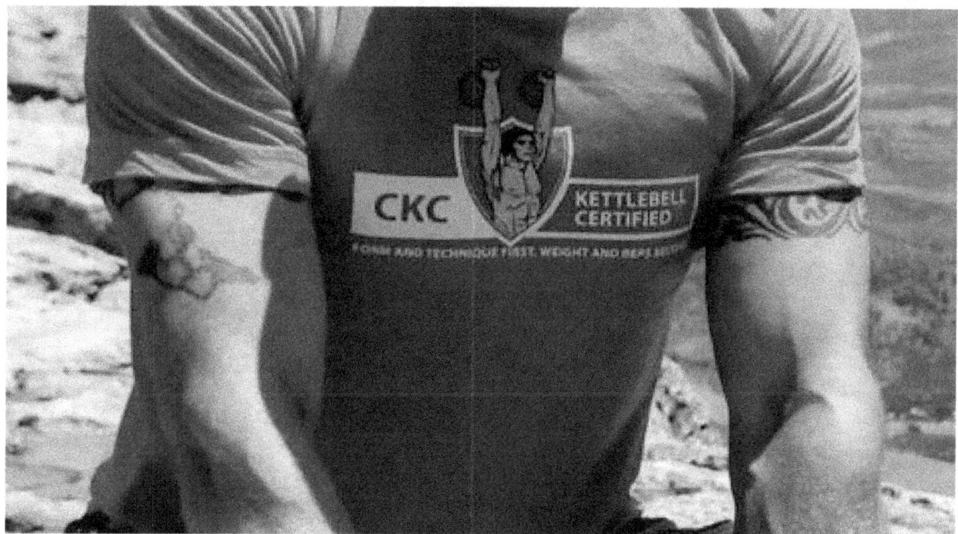

# Join Us

Join *Cavemantraining* in one of the following groups/social channels:

- Kettlebell Training 11,000+ members as of 2019
  www.facebook.com/groups/KettlebellTraining/

- Kettlebell Workout 2,500 members as of 2019
  www.facebook.com/groups/kettlebell.workout/

- Kettlebell Enthusiasts 2,500 members as of 2019
  www.facebook.com/groups/kettlebell.enthusiasts/

- Kettlebell Training on Reddit
  www.reddit.com/r/kettlebell_training

- Cavemantraining on Pinterest
  pinterest.com/Cavemantraining

- Cavemantraining on YouTube
  youtube.com/Cavemantraining

- Cavemantraining on Facebook
  www.facebook.com/caveman.training/

# Thank You

I would like to thank you for your purchase and I truly hope to hear or see you during your kettlebell journey, whether online or offline. If anything in this book has helped you in any way I'm always happy to hear about it. I have a passion for kettlebells but more so for bringing that knowledge across so that others can improve their lives, whether that is through gaining strength, cardio, flexibility, or confidence.

On the flip-side, I have done my best to provide you with the best instructions, but I also know that nothing is perfect, if there is something that you think can be improved I would love to hear about it. me@tacofleur.com

Huge thanks to my wife, son, and French bulldog for always being there for me, I could not have done this without any of you.

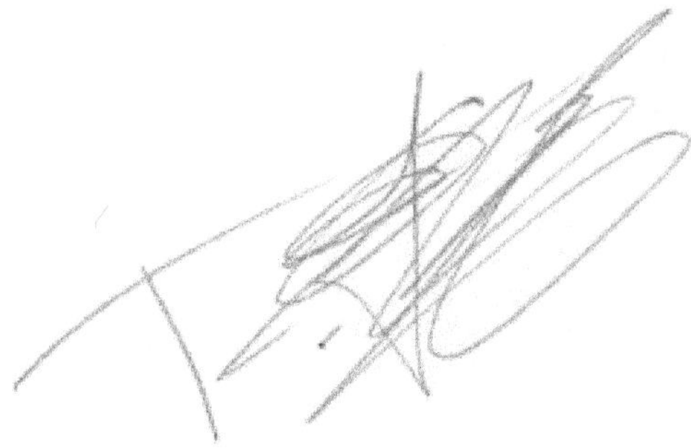